Calcium

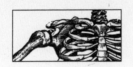

Calcium

Nature's Versatile Mineral

Bonnie Bruce, DPH, MPH, R.D.,

and

Gene Spiller, Ph.D., CNS

AVERY

a member of

Penguin Putnam Inc.

New York

Every effort has been made to ensure that the information contained in this book is complete and accurate. However, neither the publisher nor the author is engaged in rendering professional advice or services to the individual reader. The ideas, procedures, and suggestions contained in this book are not intended as a substitute for consulting with your physician. All matters regarding your health require medical supervision. Neither the author nor the publisher shall be liable or responsible for any loss, injury, or damage allegedly arising from any information or suggestion in this book.

Most Avery books are available at special quantity discounts for bulk purchase for sales promotions, premiums, fund-raising, and educational needs. Special books or book excerpts also can be created to fit specific needs. For details, write Putnam Special Markets, 375 Hudson Street, New York, NY 10014.

Avery
a member of
Penguin Putnam Inc.
375 Hudson Street
New York, NY 10014
www.penguinputnam.com

Library of Congress Cataloging-in-Publication Data

Bruce, Bonnie.
Calcium : nature's versatile mineral / Bonnie Bruce and Gene Spiller.
p.   cm.
Includes bibliographical references and index.
ISBN 1-58333-058-5
1. Calcium in the body.   2. Calcium in human nutrition.   I. Spiller, Gene A.   II. Title.
QP535.C2 B78   2000   00-035544
612.3'924—dc21

Printed in the United States of America
10 9 8 7 6 5 4 3 2

Book design by Tanya Maiboroda

Acknowledgments

MANY PEOPLE—too many to be mentioned individually—have contributed to our present knowledge of calcium and its many roles in the human body. It is because of their work that this book was made possible. Many of them had a vision that went beyond their time, which led them to discover that calcium was much more than a builder of bones.

We are thankful to our agent Georgia Hughes and to our editors Dara Stewart and Carol Rosenberg—to Dara for her advice during the early conceptual stages of this book and to Carol for her fine editing of the manuscript.

Bonnie Bruce
Gene A. Spiller
Los Altos, California

Contents

Introduction

❦

You are about to discover a whole new way of thinking about calcium. For much too long, this marvelous mineral has been sheltered within the world of bones and teeth—a centuries-old, tradition-bound connection. However, without the power of calcium, we would not have the vigor and vitality that make life worth living. In fact, since very few bodily activities escape calcium's power, a world without calcium would be a world without life.

Calcium has finally begun to emerge from its shelter. Its link to disease prevention and its role in sustaining life have become a focus of both scientific and media attention. Scientific research has uncovered a mountain of facts about calcium, and much of it goes beyond our traditional thoughts about this mineral.

Calcium: Nature's Versatile Mineral is about the practical and sometimes surprising effects that this mineral has on the human body. We wrote this book in response to the numerous comments and questions we've received over the years from students, subjects in our studies, the media, and colleagues. Also, positive results from our long-term research study on the effects of calcium supplementation on bone health in postmenopausal women further sparked our interest in sharing information about this essential nutrient with the public. So, if you've heard spates of this and bits of that about calcium and have questions of your own, this book will provide you with answers and clear up any misinformation you may have heard. It is designed to present an accurate, balanced, and interesting portrayal of the complex nature of this essential mineral. It will teach you about calcium's main functions in your body and the key players that affect those functions—both favorably and unfavorably.

This book opens with a close look at calcium's history and its widespread presence in our lives. Then, it moves on to cover the lesser-known but essential life-sustaining roles of calcium in the body. This sets the stage for clarifying the complex nature of bone and dental health and calcium's inextricable connection to osteoporosis—a disease of thinning bones. Then, we move on to reveal the more contemporary health issues surrounding calcium, including its links to heart disease, cancer, kidney stones, premenstrual syndrome, and breast cancer.

Following this, you'll learn that calcium doesn't function in isolation—nature has decreed that calcium work together with other nutrients. You'll also learn how some common nutrients and the environment within the body may impact or enhance calcium's functions. Then, the new way scientists are viewing the standards for nutrients and the newly revised recommendations for calcium intake are provided within the context of calcium needs from conception through the senior years. We examine the current recommendations for calcium intake relative to practical issues of calcium's availability to the body. And, as much as a great push is on for people to increase their intakes of calcium, the potential consequences of getting too much of this mineral is also covered.

Following an examination of traditional and other less modern calcium sources, we present a distinctive "calcium counter" aimed at helping you get the most calcium power from your food. It helps you to identify calcium sources not just by how much calcium is in them, but by teaching you how to pack as much calcium as possible into your diet to meet your needs, while being economical about calories. When it is not possible to obtain your complete calcium requirements from food, the next option is calcium in a tablet. Unscrambling the calcium-supplement puzzle is the aim of the last chapter. For those who wish to dig deeper into the various realms of calcium, additional sources are provided in the Reference section.

Calcium: Nature's Versatile Mineral will give everyone who is interested in good health or who is trying to follow his or her healthcare professional's advice a rich background and many pathways to reap the benefits of calcium's power. Everyone who reads this book will have a new appreciation and respect for the diverse and essential roles that this mineral plays in the body. Get started now to find out how you can get enough calcium without getting too much, how much at risk you may be for calcium-related health problems, and how simple it will be to take steps toward being calcium-savvy. Find out if you're doing all you can to get enough calcium and the most calcium power possible!

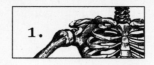

Calcium and Its History

❧

Like all minerals, calcium originates from the earth. It is the fifth most bountiful mineral on our planet and is found in most soils where plants grow and in most bodies of water. Because the human body and other life forms cannot manufacture calcium, it must be obtained from outside sources, such as foods and beverages. Calcium is the most abundant mineral in the human body, followed by phosphorus, and totals about two to three pounds by weight in the average adult. Virtually every plant and animal cell contains some calcium. Essentially, without calcium, there would be no life as we know it.

In its most basic form, calcium is a silvery-white, moderately hard metallic atom, and is among the most chemically active of all the minerals. It combines readily with numerous other elements to form chemical compounds called *salts*. Calcium salts, such as calcium phosphate, are necessary for proper growth and for the regulation of many chemical reactions that take place in the human body. By nature's design, calcium is commonly bound with other elements, such as carbon, hydrogen, oxygen, or chlorine. For example, one of the more familiar calcium-containing compounds is calcium carbonate, which is a common calcium supplement.

Calcium's Widespread Presence

Calcium is present in nearly all aspects of life. It is found in the human body, in foods, and is widespread in our daily environments. Many of us are most familiar with calcium's presence in our bones and teeth. This form of calcium is known as calcium phosphate. The next most familiar forms are calcium lactate and calcium sulfate, which are found in dairy foods, such as yogurt, cheese, and milk. Less well recognized by some people is that there is a large variety of vegetables that contain an abundance of calcium.

Few of us probably consciously think about the other numerous and diverse ways in which calcium appears in our daily lives. Without being aware of it, we likely come into contact with some form of calcium almost every day. Whenever we handle an eggshell or a seashell, drink "hard" (calcium-rich) water, see a ring around a bath tub, or wear a string of pearls, calcium is present.

Covering large regions of the earth, in many places to depths of thousands of feet beneath the surface, is limestone—made of calcium carbonate. The famous White Cliffs of Dover in England were formed from this calcium salt. In ancient Rome, limestone made up part of the mortar, or binding material, used in the building of that city. Limestone itself is thought by some to be the forerunner of plaster and Plaster of Paris. The breathtaking tropical coral reefs are made largely of calcium, and the beautiful architecture of the stalactites and stalagmites in caves were created by calcium-rich water that had dripped and hardened over centuries. Another earthly and ancient calcium-containing combination—in this case with almost equal amounts of calcium carbonate and magnesium carbonate—is dolomite. When the elements in dolomite are altered chemically, it becomes the very hard, smooth stone called marble.

Even less thought about may be the commercial use of calcium. To melt snow and ice and to keep dust from rising on roads, calcium chloride is applied. In medical settings, a calcium compound is used by blood banks to regulate blood clotting. Calcium propionate, a naturally occurring preservative, is added to some breads and other bakery products to lengthen the shelf life. Even some window glass and wall plaster contain some calcium. In our gardens, some fertilizers that enrich depleted soils are made from calcium phosphate. Have you ever been in the "limelight"? This expression originated from an early type of stage light derived from a form of calcium that produced brilliant illumination when heated. Ordinary white classroom chalk, some made from tiny seashells, is a type of fine-grained limestone. In fact, the term calcium and the word chalk are ultimately derived from the Latin word *calx*.

Calcium—One of the Oldest Known Nutrients

Calcium was among the first minerals to be recognized as being needed by humans for health and survival. It is one of the most important biologically active nutrients that the body requires in relatively large quantities on a daily basis. In its many chemical forms, calcium supports life in a wide variety of essential ways.

Despite calcium's numerous vital biological functions, many scientific advances in calcium nutrition did not take place until the twentieth century. This is because some calcium-related activities need only trace amounts of the mineral, and these actions could not be determined until chemical methods to analyze these trace amounts were developed.

Calcium's Ancient Links to Health

During the pre-scientific era of nutrition, ancient civilizations had been able to figure out ways, usually fortuitously, to satisfy their nutrient needs without knowing about nutrients. Although early civilizations did not have the scientific means to pinpoint what was responsible for the health benefits they attributed to certain foods, calcium's importance has been connected with dietary intake for many thousands of years. For example, the condition of having brittle and fragile bones, now associated with one of the most common age-related bone diseases, osteoporosis, has been recognized for millennia. More than two thousand years ago, after a brutal battle, a Greek historian had observed that the skull bones of one group of dead soldiers were hard and strong, while the bones of the other group were soft and fragile. He attributed the differences between their skulls to the headpieces worn by the soldiers with the weakened skulls. He speculated that their head coverings, which they wore all the time, apparently had prevented them from getting proper sun exposure. Since then, we have been able to pinpoint this type of bone degeneration specifically to a vitamin D deficiency. However, it is significant how his incidental observation was related to the functioning of calcium, since without vitamin D, the body cannot absorb calcium. Though the historian could not have known that a lack of calcium ultimately caused the soft, fragile bones, the information he had gathered and the connections he had made helped future scientists in their quest for knowledge about calcium.

Several other groups of people, largely by accident, also made connections between certain foods and skeletal health. For example, Asian and Middle Eastern cultures observed that those who increased their intake of ground dried bones had stronger skeletons. Native Americans and the people of Mexico speculated that those who ate corn tortillas with their meals had stronger bones. Now, corn itself doesn't contain any calcium, but when tortillas are traditionally made, the corn is first soaked in limewater—which contains calcium—to remove the corn's hard coating. Also, when a limestone mortar and pestle was used to grind the corn, calcium was inadvertently added to the cornmeal.

Pioneers in Calcium Research

In the early 1800s, Sir Humphry Davy, a British chemist and inventor of the miner's safety lamp, was first to discover that calcium was a distinct and special chemical element. At roughly the same time, a Swedish chemist had determined by analysis the calcium and phosphorus content of bones. By the mid-1800s, researchers made the initial scientific connection between nutrition and calcium. A Swiss physician found that the bones of pigeons fed a calcium-deficient diet did not form properly. When he added calcium to their diets, bone development improved. He further confirmed his findings by conducting similar experiments with different animal species.

By the early 1900s, several scientists had demonstrated that calcium is essential for the survival of all animals. However, the scientific community was still unconvinced about the strength of the relationship between calcium and bone health. Even into the mid-1900s, the prevailing medical opinion held that calcium had nothing to do with osteoporosis, although we now know that calcium offers some protection against the disease. (See Chapter 4 for more information about osteoporosis and calcium.)

Some Final Words

Since its early beginnings, scientific understanding about calcium has expanded tremendously. More and more scientists are turning their attention to this essential mineral, and the totality of what is known about calcium continues to increase virtually every day. In only the past three decades, work in calcium nutrition has intensified with milestones being marked in the understanding of calcium's importance in human growth, development, health, and most recently, as a potentially strong link in disease prevention.

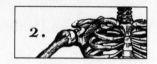

2.

Calcium's Metabolic Functions

❧

CALCIUM performs many of the body's most important life-sustaining functions, like helping to regulate muscle contraction, which includes the heartbeat. The calcium our bodies need is obtained from two sources: the intake of calcium-rich foods and the nearly limitless supply of calcium that is stored in our skeletons. Most healthy adults absorb about 30 percent of their daily dietary calcium, while other age groups, in keeping with their bodies' needs, absorb different amounts of this mineral. (See Chapter 7 for more information on calcium absorption.) In the daily course of the thousands of chemical reactions that go on in the human body, some calcium is normally lost. It is partly eliminated through the intestinal tract in the feces, and a smaller amount is excreted by the kidneys through the urine. An even smaller amount is lost through perspiration. Because the body normally loses some of its calcium, there are several mechanisms by which it maintains a constant supply of this mineral to meet its demands.

Calcium in the Body

Calcium is found in virtually every cell, tissue, and organ of the body. There are very few major biological activities that don't involve calcium's powerful and pervasive presence. Of all the elements in the human body, calcium ranks fifth in abundance. It is surpassed only by carbon, hydrogen, oxygen, and nitrogen and represents over half of the body's total mineral content. Nearly 99 percent of the body's calcium is stored in the skeleton and about 1 percent is in the teeth. The remaining tiny fraction is found in the body's fluid compartments and is referred to as *blood calcium*.

Blood Calcium

The blood calcium that circulates in the bloodstream and in the spaces between the cells is called *extracellular* calcium; the calcium found inside the cells is called *intracellular* calcium. Part of the blood calcium is present as highly active, positively charged calcium ions. These participate in the control of muscle contraction, blood clotting, nerve impulse transmission, hormone secretion, and the activation of some enzymes. The rest of the calcium found in blood is bound to proteins and helps deliver signals to the insides of the cells. It is some of these signals that are involved in helping to regulate blood pressure.

The Constancy of Blood Calcium

Because of the body's essential need for blood calcium, one of its highest priorities is to insure that its level is maintained at a precise concentration. Specialized, built-in physiological mechanisms, such as hormonal secretions and increased intestinal absorption, are activated whenever an imbalance is detected.

Over a twenty-four-hour period, blood calcium remains within a narrow range, with a very minor shift around midday. The amount of blood calcium in our bodies remains relatively steady over the course of a lifetime, decreasing only slightly with age in men, but generally remaining the same in women.

The Regulation of Blood Calcium

When blood calcium levels become too high or drop too low, the concentration is governed mainly by chemical messengers called hormones. Hormones are complex chemical compounds that are manufactured by one part of the body and travel through the bloodstream to one or more specific target sites in response to a change in the body's internal environment. Their main function is to enhance or inhibit cellular activity.

There are three main hormones involved in calcium balance. When blood calcium levels fall too low, parathyroid hormone (PTH) and vitamin D (which, in this case, acts like a hormone) are activated. When blood calcium rises too high, levels of the third hormone, calcitonin, are increased to counterbalance PTH and vitamin D activities. Each of these chemical messengers in its own specific way either mobilizes or helps to mobilize one or more major body targets—the intestines, the kidneys, and/or the skeleton—to restore balance.

PTH is released by the parathyroid glands, which are embedded in the thyroid gland in the neck region. PTH is so important to the regulation of blood-calcium levels that without it, they would suddenly drop. Vitamin D is formed in the skin after exposure to the sun's ultra-violet rays through a series of biochemical reactions. It also can be obtained from a small number of foods, such as fortified milk and margarine, liver, and fatty fish. In its role as a hormone, vitamin D functions with PTH or is transported to the intestines to help restore balance. (See Chapter 6 for more information about calcium and vitamin D.)

Calcitonin is produced by the parathyroid glands. It was not discovered until the early 1960s, so less is known about it. Scientists have established that it helps to maintain blood calcium balance, but its other functions are less understood. It is thought that it also may aid in maintaining the storage of calcium in bone when dietary calcium is in short supply, but more study is needed to confirm this.

When Blood Calcium Levels Drop

When the amount of blood calcium drops below normal—a condition known as *hypocalcemia*—PTH stimulates the kidneys' production of vitamin D. In turn, vitamin D signals the intestinal tract to increase the amount of calcium that is absorbed into the bloodstream. The amount of calcium that the body absorbs may increase to several times the normal amount depending on the signals that the body sends. At the same time, PTH signals the kidneys to slow down the amount of calcium that is excreted in the urine and also triggers the bones to release some of their calcium into the bloodstream.

In the normal course of things, some withdrawal of calcium from the skeletal reservoir to replenish blood calcium occurs with regularity in most people as the body strives to maintain its physiological balance. In the short term, this activity is harmless—as long as there is enough dietary calcium to replace what is taken from the bones. Over the long term, however, with a chronic inadequate calcium intake, the calcium that is taken from the bones will not be replaced. Years may pass without knowing that this is happening. It is later in life that the consequences of years of chronic loss of calcium from the skeleton will become evident with the development of osteoporosis. This condition is discussed in Chapter 4.

When Blood Calcium Levels Rise

When blood calcium rises above normal—a condition known as *hypercalcemia*—calcitonin functions to help stop withdrawal of calcium from the skeleton and probably plays a role in returning calcium to the bones. It also helps to reduce the amount of calcium that is absorbed into the bloodstream by helping to inhibit the action of vitamin D.

Calcium's Many Metabolic Responsibilities

Blood calcium helps to trigger a tremendous number of biochemical reactions, many of which play crucial roles that enable us to perform our daily routine activities. Without the work of calcium, some of these actions would not take place, and others would not work properly.

Calcium works closely and in an orderly fashion with numerous other compounds, which also can influence the effectiveness of the biochemical reactions that take place. The following sections highlight some of the major work this mineral performs in the body. For a broader but more general overview of calcium's many metabolic roles, see the inset "The Many Metabolic Roles of Calcium" on page 13.

Calcium's Role in Blood Clotting

When we cut a finger or scrape a knee, blood calcium is one of the key elements that helps the wound to stop bleeding. Blood clotting occurs in a many-step, cascading series of reactions that involve more than a dozen compounds in which each subsequent step is initiated by the one that immediately precedes it. When the body senses that blood vessels have been broken, special blood clotting cells, called platelets, swarm to the site of the wound. Calcium is needed to activate one of the initial compounds, prothrombin, and is again needed to convert one of the final compounds, fibrinogen to fibrin, that forms the hardened, protective blood clot that stops the bleeding. Along with calcium, one of the fat-soluble vitamins, vitamin K, and the mineral magnesium are also essential nutrients that are required in the blood-clotting process.

Calcium's Role in Muscle Movement

A small amount of calcium resides within muscle cells to help govern reactions that signal the muscles to contract and relax, or to shorten and lengthen. This includes the heart muscle. Upon a signal from the brain, calcium binds to a key protein called troponin, which is needed to activate myosin and actin—two proteins found in muscle. Calcium's binding to troponin causes myosin and actin to slide back and forth across each other in the muscle cell. In turn, this causes the muscle to shorten and lengthen in response to movement. In addition to calcium, the mineral magnesium also is involved in regulating muscular contractions.

Either an elevated or a low blood-calcium level alters the signals that are sent between the nerves that govern muscular contraction. With a low blood-calcium level, the nerve signals that travel to the muscles become so vigorous that muscles move too easily and uncontrollably and go into spasms. Cramping, muscle tremors, or muscle twitching results. This condition is known as *calcium tetany*. Tetany occurs very rarely under normal circumstances. It has been seen in severely calcium-deficient pregnant women or those who have had an excess intake of phosphorus. (Excess phosphorus also causes a decrease in blood calcium.) It also has been seen to happen in women who are breastfeeding due to the mammary glands' great demand for calcium. This condition is known as *milk fever*.

When there is an elevated blood calcium level, the muscles will contract, but won't relax—a condition known as *calcium rigor*. A very high calcium intake paired with a very high vitamin D intake (which increases calcium absorption) can cause blood calcium to rise extremely high. This may lead to the calcification or excessive deposition of calcium in the bones, to the hardening of tendons and ligaments, and eventually to calcium being deposited in organs such as the kidneys and liver. The depositing of calcium in organs is rare and has been seen primarily in people who have improperly supplemented with vitamin D (see Chapter 6).

Calcium's Role in Nerve and Cell Communication

Calcium functions as an intermediary between the external and internal environments of the body's cells and within the cells themselves. As part of an essential biochemical reaction in the body, calcium activates a special protein, known as calmodulin, by binding with it. Once activated, the calcium-bound calmodulin transmits signals from the outside to the inside of the cell. These signals essentially direct actions of some proteins that are involved in the body's hormonal and nerve-signaling activities. For example, angiotensin, a blood protein that is involved in blood-pressure regulation, along with the hormones insulin and glucagon, both of which are necessary for blood-sugar control, are among the numerous substances in the body that rely, in part, on signals that originate with calcium.

Calcium's Role in Vitamin B_{12} Absorption

Calcium—along with a protein that is secreted by the stomach, called the *intrinsic factor*—helps with vitamin B_{12}'s transport across the intestinal cells. Vitamin B_{12}, one of the water-soluble vitamins, is essential for red blood cell formation and for the growth and maintenance of the myelin sheath, the covering that protects the nerve cells. This vitamin is unique among water-soluble vitamins because large amounts of it are stored in the liver, and it can take from two to twenty years for a deficiency to develop, depending on the individual. In addition, it is found only in animal foods, such as meats, fish, poultry, eggs, and calcium-rich dairy foods.

Without calcium or when there is not enough intrinsic factor due to other reasons, a vitamin B_{12} deficiency will cause an abnormal formation of red blood cells. This type of vitamin B_{12} deficiency is called a *macrocytic* or *megaloblastic anemia*. It more commonly affects people fifty years and older, because the secretion of stomach acid tends to decrease with age. A mild vitamin B_{12} deficiency typically causes no outward symptoms. But a more advanced deficiency

---

The Many Metabolic Roles of Calcium

Calcium is a prominent activator or copartner in a tremendous number of the body's vital biochemical reactions. These go on continuously from the time of conception until the time of death. The list below just scratches the surface of calcium's pervasive and powerful influences on the human body.

- Blood clotting.
- Blood pressure regulation.
- Blood sugar control.
- Communication between cells.
- Heart beating.
- Enzyme and hormone action.
- Normal cell division.
- Releasing energy from food.
- Sending nerve impulses.
- Sending signals between the inside and outside of cells.
- Skeletal muscle movement.

may result in a tingling sensation or a weakness in the arms and legs, confusion, listlessness, and/or stomach pain. The most serious form of a vitamin B$_{12}$ deficiency is a rare condition, known as *pernicious anemia,* which can be fatal if not properly treated by a health-care professional.

Some Final Words

By calcium's very pervasive nature and biological design, the majority of this mineral's vital functions in the body take place without any conscious effort. As you are reading this book, calcium is playing a role in your muscle movement—whether you are tapping your toes while you read or are moving your fingers in readiness to turn the page. Calcium helps to send the nerve signals from your brain or muscles to direct your actions, and if you happen to get a paper cut, blood calcium will help to stop the bleeding. As you learned in this chapter, many of the body's daily life-sustaining processes are affected by calcium's omnipresence in the blood and cells, the almost endless skeletal reservoir, and the remarkable ability of the body to regulate its calcium concentrations. Very few metabolic actions escape the power of calcium.

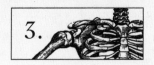

The Formation and Maintenance of Bones and Teeth

FOR MANY of us, the association between calcium and our bones and teeth has been forever fixed in our minds. This shouldn't be surprising since calcium is one of the cornerstone minerals in the architecture of these remarkable body structures. However, as powerful as the tradition holds, numerous other factors—including genetics and lifestyle habits—are influential in the ultimate growth, development, and maintenance of robust and healthy bones and teeth. These factors, some exclusive of calcium and some indirectly involving calcium, help foster or hinder the formation of a strong skeleton.

The Body's Framework

An early notion of how the body's 206 bones are arranged was illustrated in the sixteenth century by the European artist and scientist Andreas Vesalius. Through his observation as a scientist and his talent as an artist, Vesalius was able to give us an early picture of how the human body is arranged. See Figure 3.1 on page 16.

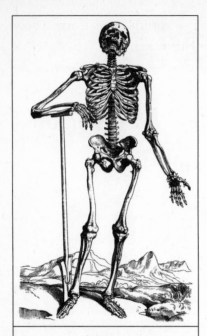

FIGURE 3.1. Andreas Vesalius, European artist and scientist, was among the first to capture in art the body's skeletal architecture.

We have since come to greatly appreciate that bones give the body its rigid structure and help to support the surrounding body tissues. Bones also help with movement by providing a solid foundation onto which muscles attach. Bones also help protect the softer, more fragile parts of the body, such as the brain (think of the skull as being like an internal bicycle helmet); the heart and lungs (think of them as being caged in by the ribs); and the spinal cord (think of it as being fenced in by the backbones). Bones are also the body's great reservoir or storage bank of calcium.

In addition to calcium, the other major minerals contained in bone are phosphorus, magnesium, and zinc. Although they are found in smaller amounts than calcium, they are of no less importance. In an average person, there is twice as much calcium as phosphorus and several hundred times more calcium than magnesium and zinc. The bones' calcium reservoir is always available to be withdrawn from the skeleton as necessary to meet the body's demands.

The Basic Construction of Bones

Each bone in the skeleton is a very complex structure made up of two different types of bone material, with calcium and phosphorus being the principal components. Eighty percent of bone is made up of a compact bone material known as cortical bone. Cortical bone fills the shafts of the leg and arm bones, as well as forming a thin covering on the outer surfaces of most bones. It is the harder of the two kinds of bone tissue. The second type of bone is a more porous, lacey-like tissue called trabecular or spongy bone. It fills the ends of the hollow cylinders of the arm and leg bones and also makes up the segments of the spinal column, called vertebrae.

Along the center portion of the bone is the marrow cavity. This is where the production of red blood cells, which are needed for carrying oxygen throughout the body; white blood cells, which are important components of the immune system; and blood platelets, which are essential to blood clotting, takes place. See Figure 3.2 below.

Filling the Calcium Reservoir

Many people think of bones as being similar to rocks—hard, solid, and inert. But the skeleton is highly active and is in constant metabolic motion. During every second of life and keeping with the metabolic demands of the body, some calcium is being withdrawn from the bones and some is being replaced. Our bones are in such a constant flux of being broken down and rebuilt day after day—a

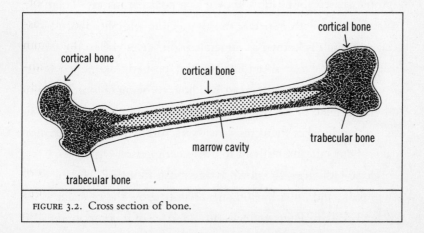

FIGURE 3.2. Cross section of bone.

process called bone remodeling—that about every five years, our bodies have essentially built entirely new skeletons.

At different stages of life, in normal, healthy people, the amount of bone that is being built relative to the amount that is being broken down varies. Until about the time we reach our mid-twenties, we are building more bone and depositing more calcium into them than what is being dismantled or withdrawn, such that the skeleton grows in size and increases in strength. From our mid-twenties to about our mid-forties, under normal circumstances and with an adequate calcium intake, the bone remodeling process is balanced—that is, we are rebuilding and dismantling bone at about the same rate. However, once we pass our forties, we begin to lose more bone than we gain. The extent to which we lose more than we gain depends on many factors, not the least of which is the lifetime intake of calcium.

Calcium's Role in Bone Building

Although there are two different kinds of bone material, all bone originates the same as the rest of the body—as the union between individual cells from our parents. The transformations that result from this unification eventually produce the unique structure and design of our calcium-rich bones. To build bone, cells first lay down a protein-based foundation known as a collagen matrix. Then, the matrix is filled with minerals, mostly calcium and phosphorus. This process, which is known as mineralization, gives rise to the typical strong nature of our skeletons. Healthy, properly developed bones are characteristically resistant to bending, to being compressed, and to being broken or fractured. The collagen matrix gives bones their strength and makes them resistant to fracture, while mineralization makes them stiff and resistant to being compressed.

Bone-building cells known as osteoblasts (think of "blasting off") use proteins and other building materials to grow the crystalline-like collagen matrix. Then minerals, in the form of a compound called hydroxyapatite, containing mostly calcium and phosphorus, attach to the fibrous network. In the finished product, hydroxyapatite makes up about two-thirds of our bones by weight.

Bone Formation and Pregnancy

The initial changes signaling the growth of the skeleton begin as early as the second week of pregnancy, but the major amount of bone mineralization in an unborn child occurs during the last three months of fetal life. A healthy infant is born with its basic skeletal structure, although its skeleton will continue to grow and strengthen into early adulthood.

For bones to form properly during early pregnancy, a woman must have an adequate intake of calories and protein. This provides the foundation for the protein-based collagen matrix on which minerals will be laid down. To lay down the minerals, an ample supply of calcium and phosphorus throughout pregnancy and early infancy is required.

Bone Formation During the Growing Years

The skeleton accrues the greatest amount of calcium between the ages of ten and twenty. This period of mineralization accounts for almost half the total amount of calcium in bone that we will have as adults. The most important time period for new bone development and mineralization is when boys and girls begin their growth spurts in the years surrounding puberty. This is when their bodies begin to produce reproductive hormones—principally estrogen and progesterone in girls; testosterone in boys—which are powerful protectors and builders of bone. During this period, proper nutrition and weight-bearing exercise are both very important factors to help ensure strong, healthy bones.

Calcium intake appears to be especially important during puberty. For girls in particular, it appears that adequate calcium is especially crucial during the two years before they begin menstruation. Fortunately, this period appears to coincide with one of the few times during the lifecycle when adequate calcium is normally consumed.

The skeleton continues to form and develop until, on average, growth in length stops in girls by about age eighteen and in boys by about age twenty. Although final bone length is achieved by the time we reach early adulthood, the accumulation of calcium in the bones and the hardening of the bones continues until about age thirty-five. This is when we achieve our peak bone mass. Maximizing the amount of bone that we develop—that is, our peak bone mass—is believed to be a significant factor in later susceptibility to degenerative bone disease. Bones are their most dense and at their strongest during this period of life. When peak bone mass has been reached, the calcium content of the skeleton will have increased from about 30 grams (about one ounce) at birth to about an average of 1,200 grams—close to 3 pounds—in an adult (see Figure 3.3 below.).

The amount of bone mass that will ultimately develop differs

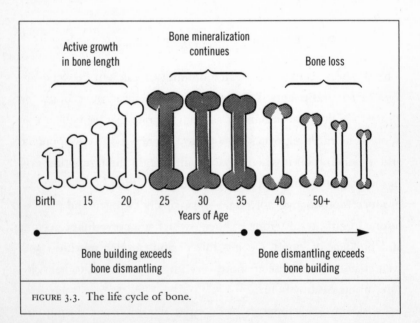

FIGURE 3.3. The life cycle of bone.

between men and women. Typically, men will have almost a third-greater bone mass than women. This is due in large part to their larger body size, which gives them an advantage as they age—they will have more calcium to spare than women. This may help to explain why men have a lesser tendency to develop age-related bone disorders.

Teeth—The Hardest Body Part

Our teeth make up the other major class of calcium-rich tissue in the body. Tooth enamel is composed largely of calcium and phosphorus and is remarkably resistant to wear and tear. It has been estimated that with good care, properly developed teeth will outlast the maximum human life span. Theoretically, given good genes and good health, we should be able to live for about 120 years, but strong teeth can last easily for 200 years.

Tooth Function and Structure

Teeth enable us to extract the robust and delicate flavors of food through their grinding and crushing actions. More important, they also help to break down food particles to more manageable sizes for digestion. Life without teeth would mean meals without crunchy, texture-rich foods or any foods that require us to chew. Well-developed, healthy teeth and a strong jaw structure—neither of which would develop properly without calcium—are needed to help get the most enjoyment and benefit from eating.

Each tooth is composed of several major parts, of which the most visible to the eye is the enamel on the surface of the tooth. The enamel, dentin, and cementum are the three mineralized parts of the tooth, which encase the nerve or pulp of the tooth—the only part of the tooth that contains living cells. Surrounding the teeth are periodontal tissues, which include the gums and the bones that help hold the teeth in place.

Tooth Formation and Development

We all grow two sets of teeth. The first set, the primary teeth—also called baby, deciduous, or milk teeth—begin to form during the first few months of fetal life, but usually do not emerge from the gums until about the second half of the first year of life or sometime later. Children lose this first set of teeth in early childhood. Permanent teeth can continue to form and develop through adolescence. By the time adulthood is reached, most of us have twenty-eight to thirty-two permanent teeth.

A poor diet, with too little calcium and vitamin D, can adversely affect tooth formation and development. If there are nutrient deficiencies during tooth development, tooth eruption may be delayed, tooth size and shape may be affected, and teeth may become crowded together in a jaw bone that has not developed properly. Small amounts of the mineral fluoride are also essential for proper tooth formation, to help strengthen teeth, and to help protect against tooth decay. However, exposure to excessive amounts of fluoride during tooth development will cause discoloration of tooth enamel, a condition known as *mottling*. There is little risk of getting toxic amounts of fluoride from the diet (all diets contain some fluoride, with tea and fish being especially good sources) or from using fluoridated tooth products. Even when the additional fluoride intake from municipal drinking water (about half of the drinking water in the United States is fluoridated) is considered, that amount is felt to be safe. Excessive exposure, which has resulted in serious cases of mottling, have been reported in communities only where the public water system failed and fluoride concentrations reached inordinate amounts.

The Calcium in Teeth

In contrast to the highly active skeletal bone tissue, which is continuously being dismantled and rebuilt, teeth are relatively inert. Once tooth formation and development are completed, little dismantling and rebuilding occurs. Although calcium is a major component of tooth structure, little or none of this mineral is available from the teeth to help meet the body's metabolic demands for calcium. On the other hand, the bones that support the teeth are similar to the rest of the bones in the body. They are just as likely to be candidates for providing calcium, if needed. Bones surrounding the teeth, or the jawbone, will become weakened when excess calcium has been withdrawn from them without adequate dietary replenishment.

The Impact of Genes on Bone Formation

The primary influence in bone development comes from our genetic backgrounds. It has been estimated that about three-fourths of what determines how our bones will grow and how strong they will be is decided by genetic factors. Beyond that, it is chiefly what we do or do not do that influences whether or not healthy bones develop.

If your grandparents had robust bones, there's a good chance that you also will have good, strong bones. Studies involving mothers and daughters suggest that the stronger your family's bone structure, the better your chances will be that your bones will be strong. For example, we have seen that young girls whose mothers had osteoporosis had less bone mass than daughters of mothers with healthy, strong bones.

The amount of bone we will form is also, in part, decided by our ethnic backgrounds. Black and Hispanic people tend to develop larger bones with greater bone mass than do Caucasians and Asians. Caucasians and Asians typically have lighter, more delicate bone structures. Within these observations, however, it is important to remember that there are wide variations due to individual differences.

Little can be done about our genetic histories, but we do have some control over a number of nutrition and lifestyle factors, outlined in the following section.

Calcium and Other Factors That Affect Bone and Tooth Formation

It is well known by most people that without sufficient calcium, neither bones nor teeth will develop optimally or become as strong as they maximally could. And although calcium and phosphorus are major minerals in bone formation, other compounds produced by the body like parathyroid hormone and vitamin D, discussed in Chapter 2, also play crucial roles. In bone formation, additional minerals, like magnesium, zinc, and the already mentioned fluoride, plus some other nutrients interactively or collectively function in the bone-building process. For tooth formation, calcium and phosphorus are also the major minerals involved, but additional nutrients are needed as well. For example, vitamin A is essential for proper formation of tooth enamel; vitamin C is needed for the formation of dentin—the bone-like material that composes the principal mass of a tooth found under the enamel; vitamin D is needed for growth, appropriate jawbone formation, and tooth mineralization; and fluoride is important for protection against dental cavity formation. However, bone and tooth formation and maintenance are not dependent solely on nutrition. Lifestyle behaviors like exercise, smoking, and even dieting can have an impact.

Physical Activity

When it comes to the benefits of weight-bearing exercise on skeletal growth and maintenance, no saying is more incisive than "use it or lose it." Having strong, robust bones in large part depends on being physically active. Regular weight-bearing physical activity appears to be especially important for children during the growing years when minerals are being deposited into the bones. Newer research suggests that it may be even more important than previously thought in helping to preserve bone mass as we age. Weight-bearing activities trigger bone-building cellular activity that in turn prompts calcium to be deposited into bone.

The Negative Effects of Too Little Exercise Being physically active is so important to skeletal health that bones, as well as our muscles, begin to lose their strength almost immediately upon becoming inactive. By studying astronauts who have spent time in zero gravity, we have seen how quickly muscles and bones begin to lose their strength. When astronauts enter space and leave the forces of the earth's gravity, they become weightless. From the first day of weightlessness, they begin to lose calcium from their bodies. After about three months in space, one study showed that there was a 2.5 percent loss of calcium from bone. Similar results have been observed in people who have become wheelchair bound, bedridden, or otherwise immobilized. This applies to young people as well as to older individuals. Young adults in their twenties have been found to lose as much as one percent of their bone for each week that they are bedridden.

Active, exercised bones are more robust and mineral-laden than those that are inactive and not exercised. To maximize bone formation and strength and to maintain their robustness, bones need regular weight-bearing physical activity. This includes walking, dancing, tennis, skiing, jogging, or weight-lifting. One university study demonstrated that women who rode a stationary bike for thirty minutes, three to four times a week, actually increased the amount of bone in their spines by 3.5 percent. Swimming is also thought to be beneficial, although it is not considered a weight-bearing activity. This is because similar biochemical responses that are stimulated by the muscle during swimming also favor the building of bone. In addition, even heavy housework, like vacuuming, heavy manual gardening, or shoveling snow, is good for the bones (and muscles, too).

The Negative Effects of Too Much Exercise Just as being sedentary is detrimental to the bones, so is an excess amount of exercising. For most of us, exercising too much is not a problem. There are some young female athletes, however, who exercise to such an extent that their bodies consequently cease to produce the female hormones, estrogen and progesterone. They stop menstruating and suffer from a condition known as *athletic amenorrhea*—loss of menstruation due to excessive exercise.

When menstruation ceases due to diminished hormone production, the bone remodeling process is impaired, and more calcium is lost from bone than is deposited into it. Athletic amenorrhea is common in female long-distance runners and ballet dancers—that is, in professions or sports where the customary practice is to rigidly control body weight. But any young adult woman, whether or not she's athletic, whose periods cease for six consecutive months may experience a significant loss of calcium from her bones. It is the diminished production of female hormones that is thought to be responsible for this bone damage.

Athletic amenorrhea is typically accompanied by a very poor diet, which contributes to the negative skeletal effects. These women's dietary patterns are usually very low in calories and calcium. Some may consume less than a thousand calories a day, with only 600 to 800 milligrams per day of calcium when they should be getting 1,000 to 1,300 milligrams of calcium per day (see Chapter 8).

With a deficient dietary calcium intake and the loss of their protective female hormones, the body begins to withdraw calcium from the skeleton to meet the metabolic demands of the body. Even more worrisome, athletic amenorrhea generally occurs in young women during the years when they are in the process of accumulating calcium in their bones to last them for the rest of their lives. At this time of great calcium need, young women are getting too little calcium, which may be setting the stage for osteoporosis in later years (see Chapter 4).

Extreme or Chronic Weight-Loss Dieting

With special reference to females—young women in particular—the extremely high cultural value American society places on being thin forces them to struggle to be at a body weight or have a body shape that is often unrealistic or impossible to obtain. Trying to win this often losing battle not only potentially jeopardizes the integrity of their bones, but also can have adverse effects on their health.

Extreme calorie restriction—following a diet that provides less than 1,000 calories per day—by itself even without excessive exercise also can contribute to bone loss. Most often undertaken for the purposes of weight loss, this level of calorie intake is almost universally calcium deficient and nearly always lacking in many other nutrients, including those needed for bone. For example, Karlene, a twenty-one-year-old student was a typical example of the one in four of Americans who is on a diet to lose weight at any given time. Although Karlene wasn't overweight, she was determined to lose five pounds, because she felt that she should be thinner and that her body should be shaped differently. During a class discussion, Karlene shared some of her experiences with low-calorie dieting in repeated attempts to lose those stubborn five pounds. She reported that when she wasn't dieting, she normally consumed a typical American diet, which was too low in calcium. And, when she was dieting, she always found herself feeling tired and irritable and suffered from frequent headaches. In general, she felt unwell whenever she was dieting.

The effects Karlene experienced generally happen to people whenever they severely reduce their calorie intake. The body senses the calorie deprivation, and it adapts by assuming what is called a *survival* or *starvation mode*. This is because the body's top priority is to meet its needs for energy—which it normally does from the calories it receives from the regular intake of food. When it is deprived of energy, the body slows the rate at which it burns calories—to save energy for vital life-sustaining activities, such as maintaining heart and lung function. Consequently, we tend to feel tired or low in energy and may even experience headaches. After a few days of continued caloric deprivation, the body then begins to break down protein from muscle tissue to supply the body with energy, first getting its needs met from the least essential muscles of the body. It also begins to use some byproducts of fat metabolism to fuel the brain and central nervous system, which can contribute to fatigue and headaches. With prolonged, severe caloric deprivation or starvation, the body begins to dismantle protein from the body's organs, like the heart. At the same time, when it is not getting enough dietary calcium, the body extracts what it needs from the skeleton to keep the blood and cells supplied. With repeated bouts of low-calorie dieting, especially without adequate replenishment when not dieting—as in Karlene's case—bone mineralization can be adversely affected.

As a general rule of thumb, to help prevent or at least minimize some of these physiological responses, calorie levels for weight-loss diets should be no lower than 10 calories per pound of body weight per day, insuring that enough calcium-rich foods are included (see Chapter 9). A calcium supplement might also be considered (see Chapter 10).

In even more severe cases, the tragic effects of extreme calorie restriction have been clearly shown in individuals with the condition known as *anorexia nervosa*. Anorexia nervosa is a serious eating disorder characterized by self-induced starvation. To a large degree, this disorder affects predominantly young teenaged girls. Sufferers of anorexia nervosa typically eat very little and usually have extremely low bone density. They also may develop osteoporosis early on, suffering fractures in their spines during their twenties. Indeed, it has been reported that bone loss in people with anorexia can be very severe, with reductions of up to 50 percent in bone mass. A prolonged, severe calcium deficiency, especially in the presence of overall malnutrition, can be fatal. About 5 to 20 percent of people with anorexia die.

Cigarette Smoking

Cigarette smoking is as harmful to the bones and teeth as it is to the rest of the body. People who smoke have, on average, 5 to 10 percent less bone mass than nonsmokers. Premenopausal women who smoke have lower levels of the bone-building estrogen hormone compared to nonsmokers and frequently go through menopause earlier. In both men and women, cigarette smokers also may absorb less dietary calcium.

Alcohol Consumption

Moderate consumption of alcohol, such as enjoying an occasional glass of wine or a bottle of beer, does not appear to harm the bones or the way that the body handles calcium. But studies have suggested that when consumed in excess amounts and more frequently than occasionally—that is, more than one to two 5-ounce glasses of wine, one 12-ounce bottle of beer, or 1 to 2 ounces of distilled liquor a day—and without the benefit of food to help slow its absorption, the potential for negative effects on calcium and bone is increased.

Alcohol is an egocentric molecule that receives preferential treatment and gets metabolized before most other nutrients. Unlike food, alcohol does not need to be digested and is quickly absorbed intact. In the process of intestinal absorption, it blocks the intestinal transport of the B vitamins thiamin, folic acid, and vitamin B_6, which are then lost to the body. In the liver, the breakdown of alcohol requires another B vitamin, niacin, which is then no longer available for the multitude of body processes for which it is required, such as helping to release the energy from food. In addition, alcohol metabolism increases the amount of acid that is produced by the body. The more alcohol that is consumed, the more acidic the body's internal environment becomes. In turn, the skeleton, as one of the body's major acid-neutralizers, releases calcium into the bloodstream to help restore the body's balance. There is also evidence from animal studies in particular that alcohol can indirectly affect the way in which the body handles calcium by influencing the activity of vitamin D and parathyroid hormone. These changes result in inhibiting bone formation and upsetting the balance between bone building and dismantling process. Finally, alcohol causes the body to produce more urine. As a result, the kidneys excrete more calcium. And, as with smokers, many heavy drinkers are known to have poor nutritional habits that are likely to be inadequate in calcium, as well as other minerals and vitamins, particularly vitamin D. Heavy drinkers also are typically not very physically active. Thus, coupled especially with an inadequate calcium intake, chronic and excessive alcohol intake can contribute to weakened bones and set the stage for future bone loss.

Medication Use

Both prescription drugs and some common over-the-counter preparations can potentially interact with calcium. They may affect the way in which calcium functions, how calcium is excreted from the body, or how calcium affects the activity of the drug itself. A recent book for physicians on drug interactions, *Drug Interaction Facts* by D. S. Tatro, describes close to a hundred different medications with calcium interactions. Most typically, they either affect calcium function in the body or cause calcium to be excreted before it is absorbed.

Table 3.1 on page 16 presents common examples of potent calcium and drug interactions. Whenever you are prescribed a new medication, you should talk to your health-care professional about potential interactions.

Some Final Words

There are so many factors in life that influence the development of healthy strong bones and teeth that it may seem remarkable that they

TABLE 3.1. POSSIBLE INTERACTION BETWEEN CALCIUM AND SOME COMMON MEDICATIONS

General Category of Medication	Interaction	Consequence
Beta Blockers (blood pressure medications)	Calcium may decrease effectiveness of some beta blockers.	Blood pressure control may not be as effective.
Iron Salts	Decreased absorption of calcium or iron.	Iron-deficiency anemia treatment becomes ineffective.
Tetracyclines (antibiotics)	Taking calcium salts or milk products at the same time decreases absorption.	Less infection-fighting power.
Thiazide Diuretics (such as Naturetin, Diuril, Lazol, Naqua, and Aquatag)	Less calcium than normal may be excreted, causing more to be retained by the body.	Possible calcium toxicity.
Verapamil (a heart drug)	Calcium diminishes effectiveness to such a great extent that calcium salts (like calcium carbonate) have been used to treat Verapamil overdoses.	May change heart rhythm and blood pressure.

last as long as they do. Calcium's powerful influence and potent roles in bone health, its interactions with other factors, and the body's outstanding ability to regulate calcium balance are major contributors. However, to form the strongest skeleton and hardest teeth, balancing those factors over which we have control is also essential. Consuming a proper diet and exercising regularly throughout life enhances our chances of developing and maintaining healthy bones and teeth. If, throughout our lives, we include wholesome, nutritious calcium-rich foods in our diets; maintain a regular routine of weight-bearing activity, like walking, vigorous housework, and gardening; and don't smoke or drink alcohol excessively, our bones and teeth will be much more likely to become robust and capable of withstanding some of the changes that come with age.

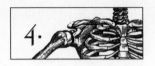

Calcium's Connection
to Osteoporosis

Osteoporosis—an age-related bone disorder that is painful, disabling, and often deforming—is a topic often associated with calcium. The word osteoporosis literally means "porous bones." This condition causes the skeleton to become extremely fragile. The bones actually become thin, porous shells due to loss of bone mineral. Severe osteoporosis, marked by bones that are easily fractured, afflicts 28 million people in the United States. Another 18 million are considered to have low bone mass, which precedes the development of osteoporosis. As baby boomers start entering their golden years, that number is expected to increase dramatically as the number of Americans over the age of sixty-five increases.

The development of osteoporosis is often mistakenly thought to result simply from a calcium deficiency. Many people are often misled or uninformed about the number of additional factors involved in its development and prevention. Fortunately, there are many steps that can be taken to help prevent or delay the onset of osteoporosis.

And, of course, calcium is one of the significant factors, but there are limits to what it can do.

The Silent Bone Disease

Osteoporosis is often called a silent disease because there usually is no warning until loss of bone mineral has become significant. It essentially results from the chronic draining of calcium and other bone-related minerals from the bones without sufficient replenishment. The skeleton gradually loses its strength usually before the disease is detected. In most people, it takes decades for osteoporosis to develop into an extremely serious debilitating condition—where the skeleton becomes so mineral-depleted that fractures occur for little or no apparent reason. Unfortunately, osteoporosis is often diagnosed after severe bone loss has occurred.

When Bone Loss Begins

Some bone loss is a natural consequence of aging. However, in some people, the loss of skeletal calcium that eventually leads to osteoporosis may begin early in life. Those at an increased risk include sufferers of anorexia nervosa, those who have lifelong histories of restrictive weight-loss dieting, and premenopausal women who have lost the ability to produce female hormones, which are known to be bone-protective, due to illness or surgery and haven't taken the proper steps to replace them.

On average, healthy adults begin to lose more bone than they form toward the end of their third decade of life. As the years progress, calcium continues to be drained at a slightly higher rate than it is replaced. Annually, in both men and women, about one-half percent to one percent of bone is lost between the ages of thirty and fifty. This loss increases with age. Without care and effort to replenish the calcium supply, by the time we reach our sixties, the loss of calcium from the skeleton can be sizable. Men may have lost, on average, 20 to 30 percent of their bone mass by their sixth decade. Women may have lost, on average, almost twice that amount—about 45 to 50 percent—mainly due to hormonal changes, which accelerate losses during the menopausal years.

When Osteoporosis Makes Itself Known

When there is a substantial loss of bone mineral, the skeleton loses its ability to structurally support the body. The first sign of osteoporosis may be a bone fracture caused by a fall that we blame on clumsiness or the dog underfoot. But the bone itself may have crumbled first, which had caused us to fall.

Fractures from osteoporosis can result from a simple movement that is too strenuous for the bone to handle—like bending over, picking up a bag full of groceries, or lifting the cat. If we could see the fractured bone, it would be thin and brittle, having had lost much of its mineral content. When it fractured, we had moved in such a way that was too much of a strain for the weakened bone, and so it crumbled.

Detecting Osteoporosis Before It's Too Late

In the past, osteoporosis has been diagnosed primarily after there has been a significant amount of bone loss, or after one or more fractures have occurred. There are now additional methods that can help detect bone loss before it becomes severe. These include special types of X-rays—one of which is the DEXA (dual X-ray absorptiometry)—which analyzes the amount of bone density at specific sites of the skeleton. There are also certain blood and urine tests that can suggest whether you may be dismantling more bone than you are building. Unfortunately, some of these tests are not done routinely. Check with your health-care professional about the availability.

Who Should be Concerned About Porous Bones?

When we ask women to tell us their top health concerns, we most often hear "breast cancer" as their ultimate greatest fear. Indeed, many of the young and middle-aged women we know seem especially concerned about breast cancer. And rightly so, since a woman's lifetime risk of breast cancer is about one in eight, and cancer is indeed a most onerous disease. (See Chapter 5 for more information on breast cancer.) In contrast, few of them express concern, if any, about osteoporosis—even given the fact that osteoporosis is the fourth leading cause of death among women after heart disease, cancer, and stroke. In addition, the average woman has a one in four chance in her lifetime of fracturing a bone due to osteoporosis. If it is a hip fracture, there is also a good chance of dying within a year from complications, such as pneumonia or blood clots.

Most of the damaging effects of osteoporosis are seen in post-menopausal women, so the emphasis surrounding this degenerative disease is primarily on women. However, men also develop this disease, although in fewer numbers. Approximately one-fifth of men over the age of sixty-five will suffer at least one fracture due to osteoporosis. This lower risk is due to several factors. In the first place, men have more bone to lose, because they typically have larger, denser skeletons and bigger frames than women do. Men also maintain higher levels of protective hormones longer into their life span than women do. The male sex hormone, testosterone, which helps the body to retain bone, is produced rather steadily into a man's seventh or eighth decade of life. Furthermore, men on the whole tend to consume more dietary calcium than women do.

Potential Signs of Osteoporosis

Because of the silent nature of osteoporosis, there are few, if any, visible warning signs during its earliest stages. However, there are some signals discussed below that might give you a clue that it may be developing.

Loosened Teeth or Gum Problems

As discussed in Chapter 3, calcium is not lost from teeth as it is from bone, but our teeth can become loosened and even fall out if the jawbone, which helps hold our teeth in place, begins to disintegrate. A weakened jawbone also may contribute to gum problems, such as inflammation or bleeding. Thus, before osteoporosis advances to the bone-fracture point, it may be your dentist detecting gum disease or loosened teeth that may be a potential early visible sign of osteoporosis, since the jawbone is one of the first bones that loses calcium.

Researchers have found that elderly women with osteoporosis had lost more teeth than women who had healthier bones. Thus, any unusual or unexpected tooth loss, loose teeth, or loss of bone from the jaw should send up a red flag. In such a case, a call to your health-care specialist is warranted.

A Hunched-Over, Deformed Back

As the severity of the loss of mineral from the backbones of the upper spine increases, the backbones collapse and flatten, resulting in compression fractures. As the number of these fractures increases, they create a classic hunched over appearance as shown in Figure 4.1 on page 37, commonly known as the dowager's hump or medically called *kyphosis*. A dowager's hump doesn't always cause pain. Indeed, some individuals may be walking around with spinal fractures with-

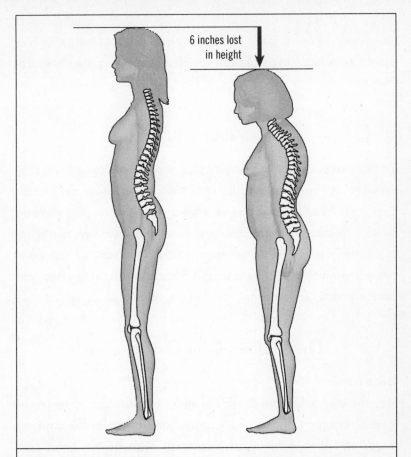

FIGURE 4.1. Young woman with normal spine (left). Older woman with dowager's hump (right).

out knowing they have a broken bone. When there is pain, it is usually a chronic, dull low backache. In severe cases, the pain can cause breathlessness, pallor, nausea, and vomiting, requiring medical treatment for the pain.

Loss of Height

As osteoporosis progresses, and as the vertebrae, or backbones, collapse and become flattened, the back loses length. In turn, we lose height and become shorter. Over the years, as osteoporosis increases in severity, a person may lose four to eight inches in height. Loss of height goes hand in hand with the development of the dowager's hump.

Chronic Bone or Back Pain

As the vertebrae lose their density, they become unable to protect the spinal nerves from pressure. This can cause excruciating and chronic back pain. In addition to loss of height, chronic back pain also may be seen together with the dowager's hump. Furthermore, any bruising or swelling around a bone or any pain in a specific area that worsens when touched may be a sign of a fracture you don't know you have, especially if you hadn't suffered any noticeable injury.

The Hallmarks of Osteoporosis

Bone fractures are the hallmarks of osteoporosis, and any part of the skeleton may be fractured, but not all fractures are caused by osteoporosis. Fractures due to osteoporosis, particularly in the advanced stages of bone deterioration, can occur without our knowledge when there is little or no stress placed on the skeleton. This is what medical experts call low-trauma fractures. An example of a low-trauma fracture would be a fracture that occurs from simply lifting a child or even from sneezing. This is in contrast to the fracture that occurs as a result of a forceful fall, such as during that whirlwind run down the ski slope or falling from a tall ladder.

Most Common Fracture Sites

The most typical kinds of fractures from osteoporosis involve the wrists, spine, and hips. The least frequent and least severe in terms of complications and long-term consequences are wrist fractures, called Colles' fractures. A fifty-year-old female has a 15 percent risk over her lifetime of suffering a fractured wrist. Fortunately, wrist fractures usually heal well, leaving virtually no limitations in movement. Fractures of the spine, called compression fractures, are most common in women fifty-five to seventy-five years old. Spinal fractures occur when weakened bones in the spine collapse and crush in on themselves. These are a common cause of severe, chronic back pain, loss of height, and the dowager's hump (see page 38).

Hip fractures are about two times more common in women than in men and occur in about one-fifth of postmenopausal women up to age eighty. After age eighty, it is estimated that up to one-half of women will have had a hip fracture. Hip fractures are perhaps the most serious of all types of fractures. The elderly are especially at risk since they tend to have less muscle and fat mass around their hips to cushion a fall. The death rates associated with hip fractures are almost one-third higher than they are for other types of fractures usually due to complications from treatment. Furthermore, they are among the top reasons the elderly end up in nursing homes. A large percentage of hip-fracture victims never fully recover their ability to walk and do not regain their independence.

What Puts Us at Risk for Osteoporosis?

Osteoporosis is not a simple disease with a singular cause. Multiple factors contribute to the likelihood of developing it, not the least of which is the role played by calcium. Conditions and lifestyle behaviors that lead to osteoporosis may be interactive, or synergistic. Many people with osteoporosis may have several risk factors, while others who develop the disease may not. Just being a woman is one of the primary factors that will put you in a higher risk group for developing osteoporosis, but there are several other factors over which most women have at least some control. The following is a discussion of the risk factors for osteoporosis, which are summarized in Figure 4.2 below.

Family History

Look at your grandparents, parents, siblings, and even your aunts and uncles—their lifelong skeletal health will give you a clue as to what you might expect for yourself. We know that genetic background is one of the determining factors in how strong our bones will be. Therefore, our chances of developing osteoporosis are increased if we have a relative with osteoporosis or one who has a history of broken bones that occurred under normal conditions or from minor falls.

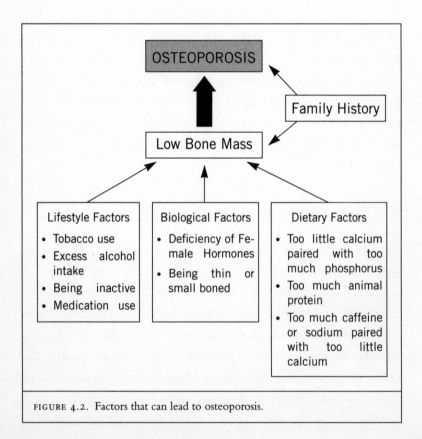

FIGURE 4.2. Factors that can lead to osteoporosis.

Being Thin or Small-Boned

Being underweight or small-boned is associated with a lower bone density than being of normal weight or being overweight. Someone who is thin or small-boned tends to have an increased possibility of developing osteoporosis, because there is a smaller stockpiling of bone mineral from which the body can draw. Actually, being overweight has been shown to be a protective factor in osteoporosis development. However, bone health should not be used as a reason to become or remain overweight—the health risks associated with having an excess amount of body fat far outweighs the protection gained against bone loss.

Dietary Imbalances

In general, the typical American diet is too high in some dietary constituents and way too low in others. This is especially true for calcium. These dietary imbalances can contribute to calcium loss from the skeleton or increase loss from the body, both of which over time can increase the risk of developing osteoporosis.

When a calcium-deficient diet is accompanied by a high protein intake—especially animal protein—and/or there is a surplus intake of phosphorus relative to calcium intake, calcium losses can be significant. Also, we have known for decades that too much sodium and too much caffeine in a diet lacking in calcium leads to calcium losses. In addition, chronic intake of too much alcohol also can increase risk of osteoporosis.

Physical Inactivity

Modern technology has created a wealth of timesaving and labor-saving devices—from the automobile to the electric knife and the can opener—all of which lead us to move our bones (and muscles) less. A physically active life is essential to healthy bones. Regular participation in weight-bearing activity stimulates bone building. Conversely, being inactive, especially with a diet lacking in calcium, causes bone dismantling to exceed bone building. Aging, coupled with inactivity, further increases bone loss. Inactivity is clearly an enemy of healthy, strong bones. (See Chapter 3 for more information on physical activity and bone-building.)

Tobacco Use

The damaging effects of smoking appear to affect virtually every organ and tissue in our bodies, including the bones. Smokers usually have less bone mass and increased risk of fractures, because hormonal activity and the body's handling of dietary calcium may be adversely affected. There is little doubt that smoking increases chances of producing a weakened skeleton, setting the stage for osteoporosis.

Presence of Medical Conditions and Chronic Use of Certain Medications

Unfortunately, some of us have illnesses that we may have inherited or acquired. Some of these can have unfavorable, long-term effects on the skeleton. There are links between bone loss and diabetes, hyperparathyroidism (a condition where too much parathyroid hormone is produced), rheumatoid arthritis, and osteoarthritis. In addition, bone loss can occur from chronic use of several common medications, many of which are used to treat these conditions. These include corticosteroids, anticoagulants, diuretics, anticonvulsants, and some psychoactive medications. (See Table 3.1 in Chapter 3 for more information concerning medication use and calcium.)

Dwindling Female Hormones

A diminished production of the female hormones—estrogen and progesterone—resulting from menopause or surgical removal of the ovaries—is strongly linked to the development of osteoporosis. The normal reduction in hormone production that occurs with menopause takes place, on average, in the fifth decade of life. By the time many women have completed menopause, about one-third of them will have lost a considerable amount of bone mass.

Female hormones are powerful bone-building and protective substances, and particularly in the years immediately following menopause, a woman may lose 10 to 20 percent of her bone mass due to their dwindling production. There is little that can be done about the natural changes that occur with age, but there are several medical treatment options that are known to help. A woman reaching menopause who is concerned about her bones should consult her health-care professional about available options.

Calcium's Role

An adequate intake of calcium over our lifetimes is one of the most important factors to help insure that we form proper bones and that they are optimally maintained. Helping to build strong bone is among the most powerful of the protective roles that calcium plays. Storing ample calcium in our bones insures a large calcium cushion to rely on when the body's bone dismantling process begins to outweigh its bone building capabilities.

Although calcium's importance in bone health cannot be overemphasized, keep in mind that osteoporosis is not a calcium-deficiency disease, per se. High intakes of calcium during adulthood, after bone has been lost, will not make up for loss of bone that has already occurred. Dietary calcium by itself will not reverse the disease. But getting enough calcium throughout adulthood may help to slow future damage to the skeleton.

Are You at Risk for Osteoporosis?

At this time, it is not medically possible to completely stop the normal bone loss that occurs with aging, but there are several things we can do to help prevent or delay the development of osteoporosis. The odds of developing osteoporosis are high, but not all of us will develop it or have it serious enough for it to become a health threat. Some factors cannot be changed, but to a large degree, we can control whether or not we get adequate dietary calcium and whether or not we are physically active. Also, we have control over other lifestyle behaviors that we know will adversely affect the skeleton.

Take a minute to see where you stand. Look over the checklist below and think about the items as they apply to you. See how they add up. The more risk factors you have, the greater chance you have of developing osteoporosis. Consider each item wisely, taking those that you can do something about most seriously.

Checklist: Are You at Risk for Osteoporosis?

Check all the items that apply to you. The more that apply to you, the higher your risk of developing osteoporosis. For those things that you can change, think seriously about taking the appropriate steps to change them.

- ☐ I am a woman.
- ☐ I have a family history of osteoporosis or have family members who have suffered fractures, particularly of the spine, hip, or wrist, not due to serious accidents.
- ☐ I am small boned or have been underweight for much of my life.

☐ My dietary calcium intake has been low for most of my life.

☐ My dietary intake of protein, especially animal protein, is or has been high.

☐ My dietary intake of sodium has been high.

☐ My dietary intake of phosphorus, relative to calcium, has been high.

☐ My caffeine intake, relative to my calcium intake, has been high.

☐ I frequently have more than one alcoholic drink.

☐ I do not or have not regularly participated in any weight-bearing activities, such as walking, jogging, weight-lifting, or playing tennis.

☐ I smoke cigarettes.

☐ I have one or more medical conditions, such as diabetes, hyper-parathyroidism, rheumatoid arthritis, or osteoarthritis, which are linked to bone loss.

☐ I take or have taken for six months or more medications, such as corticosteroids, anticoagulants, diuretics, or anticonvulsants, that can potentially increase loss of calcium from bone.

☐ I am menopausal or had my ovaries surgically removed before age fifty and have not done anything about my loss of female hormones.

Some Final Words

Even though women are at much higher risk for osteoporosis than men are, both sexes should be consciously aware of factors that can affect their chances of developing this all too prevalent disease. The sooner they take action to help protect the skeleton, the greater the benefit will be. Even when osteoporosis is present, it's never too late to start taking action. If you don't pay attention to what you are do-ing or not doing when it comes to your bone health, and calcium is chronically being lost from the skeleton without being replaced, you may end up fracturing a bone while performing a simple everyday task. Don't let thin, porous, fragile bones become part of your life.

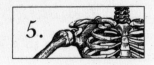

The "New" Health Benefits of Calcium

As the importance of calcium's role in nutrition and disease has become increasingly recognized, scientific interest has escalated and expanded into areas where previously calcium was given little thought. In recent years, calcium has been the center of research relative to its potential and promising roles in preventing and treating some contemporary health problems. Research regarding some of the previously known associations with calcium and disease are being confirmed, while research on some of the newly recognized protective relationships is just emerging. Some of calcium's relationships include the following:

- Regulation of blood pressure.
- Protection from colon cancer.
- Prevention of kidney stones.
- Reduction of symptoms associated with premenstrual syndrome.
- Reduced risk of breast cancer.

An Overview of High Blood Pressure and Its Relationship to Calcium

High blood pressure, or hypertension, is a major risk factor for both coronary heart disease and stroke—two of the top causes of death in the United States. Over the years, it has become evident that diet and lifestyle habits contribute to the development of high blood pressure. For example, it has been observed consistently that when different ethnic groups migrate to the United States and adopt the Western way of life, their blood pressures tend to increase. This is likely due in part to the typical Western lifestyle, which is significantly different from that in many other countries, especially non-industrialized regions. The typical Western diet is animal-based and high in fat and sodium, low in calcium and other minerals like magnesium, low in some vitamins and low in plant foods. In contrast, traditional diets of non-industrialized regions are typically high in grains, fruits, and vegetables and low in animal foods. Additionally, other components of a Western way of life also include smoking and drinking alcohol, and being sedentary, obese, and highly stressed— all of which can contribute to hypertension.

Scientists have long studied the relationship between diet and hypertension. During the past few decades, they have found that calcium, magnesium, and potassium are among the principal minerals associated with high blood pressure. In particular, several studies have shown that low calcium diets were associated with higher blood pressure, and that consumption of balanced diets that provide adequate calcium help to lower blood pressure.

About the Blood Pressure-Calcium Connection

The body's ability to regulate blood pressure is vital to life. The heart muscle is responsible for pushing the blood through the arteries, while the nervous system helps to maintain the amount of pressure in the arteries by adjusting their size and influencing the pumping action of the heart. Blood calcium is necessary for the heart muscles to contract and relax and for the nervous system to transmit its messages properly.

Studies on the Blood Pressure-Calcium Connection

The most exciting findings have come from the landmark DASH (Dietary Approaches to Stop Hypertension) study that was published in 1997 in *The New England Journal of Medicine*. These results have important implications for reducing blood pressure in the United States and for supporting the importance of a calcium-rich diet. This multi-center study compared three groups of subjects with high blood pressure—Caucasians, Hispanics, and African-Americans—who consumed different kinds of diets. Subjects on the DASH diet (a low-fat diet that included an abundance of calcium-rich dairy products, fruits, vegetables, and grains) were compared with subjects who consumed a higher fat diet that was low in calcium, but high in fruits and vegetables, and also with subjects who consumed a typical Western diet. And, to make the results more applicable to the general public, none of the subjects had to severely restrict their sodium or alcohol intake—both of which can increase blood pressure in some people. The most significant reduction in blood pressure occurred in the group of subjects eating the DASH diet. Additionally, when the results between the groups were examined separately, the DASH diet appears to be significantly helpful in lowering blood pressure in African-Americans, who have two to three times the risk over their Caucasian counterparts for high blood pressure. Furthermore, the results are especially compelling, since the DASH diet is the same type of diet that is recommended by most nutrition scientists and public health professionals.

Another special appeal of the DASH diet is that it is easy to follow. In general, for someone who needs 2,000 calories a day, eating the DASH way simply means eating 7 to 8 servings of grains with an emphasis on whole grains, 4 to 5 servings each of fruits and vegetables, and 2 to 3 servings of low-fat or fat-free, calcium-rich dairy foods each day. A serving of lean meat, fish, or poultry is limited to 6 ounces per day.

Adding more support to the blood pressure-calcium connection was a study with African-American adolescents, who are known to have a low calcium intake. This study found that increasing the calcium intake of these teens had a beneficial effect on blood pressure, which suggests that the age-related increase in blood pressure may be delayed or possibly prevented.

As it stands, the relationship between calcium and blood pressure regulation is a strong one. Research indicates that calcium is a contributor in helping to prevent hypertension, and may contribute to lowering blood pressure. However, because these studies tested diets that contain a wide variety of nutrients and other bioactive compounds naturally found in foods, rather than studying only calcium, it is likely that other dietary compounds also help to regulate blood pressure. Thus, these results do not suggest that we all should start taking calcium tablets for our blood pressure. Instead, these studies further support the importance of getting the proper amount of calcium, in addition to liberal amounts of fruits and vegetables in our daily diets.

Furthermore, it is important to remember that diet alone is not the only factor involved in blood pressure control. In addition to diet, maintaining a healthy weight for your body frame, participating in a regular routine of physical activity, not smoking, consuming moderate amounts of sodium and alcohol (if you drink at all), and managing your responses to stress through stress-management techniques are also important to blood pressure regulation.

Calcium and the Possible Prevention of Colon Cancer

In the United States, cancer of the colon is the fourth most common cancer after breast, lung, and prostate cancers, and it is the second top cause of cancer-related death. Colon cancer does not distinguish between men and women, affecting both sexes at approximately the same rate.

Since the mid-1900s, scientific reports have continued to point to a protective role for calcium in reducing the risk of developing colon cancer. One of the early observational studies linking calcium to colon cancer showed that Northern Europeans whose diets were high in fiber and fermented milk products, such as yogurt, had lower rates of colon cancer. Another large study of postmenopausal women showed that as calcium intake went up, the chances of developing colon cancer went down. Still other studies have linked lower rates of colon cancer specifically to higher intakes of dairy foods.

There is both theoretical and experimental research to support calcium's role in protection from colon cancer. Much of the evidence comes from studies of cellular growth in the colon of animals, but some human research also has suggested that calcium may interrupt cancer tumor growth. Some scientists think that the calcium that is lost through the intestinal tract in the feces binds with certain harmful, cancer-causing compounds and carries them out of the colon along with other body wastes. This interrupts the potential for these compounds to damage or irritate the colon's delicate cells and thus stop cellular irritation and stimulation of cancer cell growth. In this case, both calcium supplements and calcium-rich foods have been studied and both appear to be helpful. Results from studies suggest that when we take in enough calcium to meet or slightly exceed current recommendations, we get some protection from colon cancer. Note, however, that it is still too early in the scientific process to identify precisely what role calcium plays in the prevention of colon cancer.

Calcium and Kidney Stones

Kidney stones are a painful, debilitating condition. They are one of the oldest known medical afflictions. About 10 to 20 percent of the American population develops them at some time during their lives. Folklore and early scientific theories had often indicted calcium as the cause. The medical profession at one time believed that restricting calcium would help to prevent kidney stone formation.

The folklore and traditional thinking surrounding calcium and its association with kidney stones are based on the logical relationship that the most common type of kidney stone is composed principally of calcium that is bound with oxalic acid—known as calcium oxalate stones. Oxalic acid is a compound found in some foods, but in the case of kidney stones, some of the oxalic acid involved may be synthesized by the body. (See Chapter 7 for more information about oxalic acid.) Current research suggests that, in fact, it is not the calcium that increases the chances of forming a calcium oxalate stone in most first-time stone formers. An adequate calcium intake may, in fact, reduce risk. Researchers believe that calcium binds with the oxalic acid in a meal, so that the oxalic acid is rendered unavailable for kidney stone formation. Further, it may be the oxalic acid that plays a greater role in increasing the risk of kidney stone development partly because it takes much less oxalic acid than calcium to stimulate stone formation. When calcium intake is low, urinary excretion of oxalic acid increases, which favors kidney stone formation.

Recent long-term studies have found that both men and women who had the highest dietary calcium intakes had lower risks of developing a first time kidney stone than those with lower calcium intakes. Researchers further noted that the individuals at lower risk also had higher intakes of fluid, vitamin K, magnesium, and phosphorus, thus adding support to the notion that calcium may not be acting in isolation, but may be interacting with these other nutrients in its protective effects.

In some instances, research has shown that calcium supplements may not be as beneficial in reducing vulnerability to the formation of kidney stones as calcium-rich foods. This is because many people do not take their calcium supplements with meals—which aids the absorption of some kinds of calcium supplements. Also, the calcium found in foods occurs naturally with other nutrients or constituents in the food, which, as was suggested previously, may be needed for maximum benefit. Furthermore, some scientists think that calcium tablets may actually increase the concentration of oxalic acid (the principal partner with calcium in calcium oxalate stones), which in turn may have the opposite effect and increase the chances of kidney stone formation.

One final word of caution: Most studies have looked at prevention in people with no previous history of kidney stones. Calcium's role in risk reduction of forming recurrent stones is less clear. You should consult your health-care professional for advice.

Calcium and Premenstrual Syndrome

Nearly half of the women of childbearing age experience a cluster of widely varying uncomfortable symptoms shortly before their menstrual periods, known as premenstrual syndrome (PMS). At least one in twenty women report one or more symptoms as being so severe that they are temporarily disabled. Symptoms like cramping, nausea, bloating, backaches, or breast tenderness can be caused by physiological and hormonal changes, or may be linked to mood changes such as depression or irritability. There also can be increases in appetite and cravings for certain foods—with cravings for sweets and chocolate appearing to be particularly strong.

There is no scientific consensus about the cause of PMS, although a wide range of scientific theories and popular claims have been proposed, such as deficiencies of vitamin B$_6$, vitamin E, and zinc. But most have little scientific basis. Calcium has recently become of interest in the scientific study of PMS, and one study has suggested that it just might play a role.

Results from the recent placebo-controlled pilot study hold promise that calcium may help to make PMS symptoms less severe. Several hundred PMS sufferers, between eighteen and forty-five years old, took either a placebo (an inactive substance without calcium) or a calcium supplement in the form of an antacid that provided 1,200 milligrams of calcium per day over three monthly cycles. The study found that the group taking the calcium supplement reduced their PMS symptoms by almost half compared with the placebo group.

However, don't reach for the calcium supplements just yet. It is important to examine some flaws in this preliminary study. Typical of many studies that rely on personal perception of change, the placebo group also experienced a big improvement and a large reduction in symptoms. This makes it difficult to confirm whether or not the calcium supplement was responsible for the improvement. Also, this is only a preliminary study. Scientific proof is never based on a single report, and dietary habits or supplementation practices should never be changed based on the results of one study. This study needs to be replicated before we can conclude with certainty that calcium can improve PMS symptoms.

On the other hand, supporting these results is the well-known fact that most premenopausal women have calcium-deficient diets. Given the importance of calcium in regulating various hormones and muscle and nerve activities, it is highly conceivable that calcium may be a significant factor, and perhaps a major one, in reducing the monthly discomfort experienced by so many women. Until we know for certain, one of the best actions you can take is to make sure you are getting enough dietary calcium daily.

Calcium and Decreasing the Risk of Breast Cancer

Breast cancer is a very complicated disease that involves numerous genetic and environmental factors. Based on some of the links between diet and breast cancer, and extending the findings about calcium and colon cancer discussed on page 51, relatively recent preliminary studies with animals hint that calcium along with vitamin D may be involved in lessening the chances of cancerous cell growth in breast tissue. In these animal studies, scientists observed that a diet low in calcium and vitamin D coupled with high intakes of fat, which is typical of the Western-style diet, leads to increased growth of breast cells. When calcium and vitamin D were added to the animals' diets, cell growth did not take place.

Bear in mind that this data is very preliminary and, as such, more research—especially with humans—is needed to define calcium's role in breast cancer. This area of research does appear to be promising, however. We also need to explore the effects of calcium and other nutrients on breast cells. Since vitamin D and calcium together may be involved, it further underscores the importance of getting enough calcium as well as other nutrients in our diets.

Some Final Words

Calcium's standing as a major mineral in human nutrition has advanced considerably beyond its traditional focus on bones and teeth. Current studies and ongoing research are making it visibly clear that calcium affects our overall health and is significantly involved in some of the more compelling and debilitating diseases and conditions of modern times. Despite this growing body of evidence, coupled with the fact that the majority of us are consuming inadequate amounts of calcium, a lack of calcium may become one of the most notable nutritional deficiencies of our times.

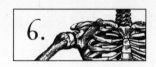

6.

Calcium's Interaction With Other Nutrients and Dietary Compounds

❦

WHEREVER calcium is found in the body, there are other nutrients or dietary compounds not classed as nutrients that function with it in interactive or synergistic ways. They can affect calcium's activity beneficially, adversely, or in both ways, depending on whether or not there are dietary deficiencies or excesses or disturbances in the body's metabolic activities. The most traditionally recognized nutrients that work in partnership with calcium are phosphorus and vitamin D. Other familiar co-workers are magnesium, zinc, and fluoride. Additionally, vitamin C and vitamin A have been shown to affect calcium's activity in the body, and recently, vitamin K has been added to the list. Even dietary fiber, the bioactive compounds phytic acid and oxalic acid, and protein play active roles in calcium nutrition.

Phosphorus—Calcium's Traditional Partner

Next to calcium, phosphorus is the second most abundant mineral in the body. Like calcium, about 150 years ago the nutritional role of phosphorus was recognized when its function in bone formation was observed. About a third of the body's phosphorus is combined with calcium as a major component of hydroxyapatite, the principal compound of bones and teeth, discussed in Chapter 3. For this reason, and because phosphorus helps with the intestinal absorption of calcium, the two minerals are usually discussed together.

In addition, like calcium, phosphorus performs other vital functions in the body that are unrelated to bone health. The phosphorus not contained in bone is distributed throughout nearly every cell of the body and participates in a wide range of the body's activities. Phosphorus is a component of DNA and RNA—the molecules that contain our genetic codes. It is central to the body's ability to work and play as part of adenosine triphosphate (ATP), a high energy compound that is a key source of energy. Phosphorus is also a vital component of the cell membrane, which controls cellular entrance and exit of molecules, including molecules of calcium.

Phosphorus is so readily abundant in our food supply that a deficiency of this mineral is rare. Meats, fish, poultry, eggs, and cheese are rich sources of phosphorus. Plant foods, like nuts, legumes, and whole grains, are also good natural sources. But phosphorus is also a very popular food additive that is used widely to improve the taste and quality of many convenience foods and cola beverages—the types of foods that tend to be the mainstay of the typical Western diet. In fact, the average American consumes nearly 50 percent more phosphorus than recommended.

Unfortunately, many phosphorus-rich convenience products are replacing some of the major calcium-containing foods, like milk, in the American diet. Of particular concern is the increasing intake of phosphoric acid-containing carbonated beverages, such as colas, by children and adolescents, especially young teenaged girls. Too many young girls, whose needs for calcium are substantial, are replacing milk with carbonated cola beverages. In general, recent national diet surveys of American adolescents have found that teens have doubled or tripled their consumption of soft drinks. As a consequence, they have cut their consumption of milk by more than 40 percent. Consequently, their low calcium and high phosphorus intakes can interfere with the body's ability to absorb calcium. In turn, bone mineral development may be impaired.

Balancing Calcium and Phosphorus Intake

Since phosphorus is abundant in meats, by its very nature a high phosphorus diet implies a high protein diet with the same downside: little or no calcium. Fortunately, phosphorus also is abundant in calcium-rich foods. Some scientists believe that there is a proper ratio of phosphorus to calcium that will help optimize calcium absorption. For example, calcium-rich dairy foods and some calcium-rich plants provide almost optimum ratios.

Table 6.1 on page 59 shows the calcium to phosphorus ratio of some common foods. To figure out the calcium to phosphorus ratio of a food that is not listed, it can be calculated from any food composition table like those found in the back of most nutrition textbooks. First, divide the amount of calcium in milligrams by the amount of phosphorus in milligrams then use the number one as the base of the ratio. This will be the ratio for calcium. Put a colon after the number one and then use the number you got for phosphorus to display the ratio. For example, if a food contains 500 milligrams of calcium and 1,000 milligrams of phosphorus, the calcium to phosphorus ratio would be 1:2. The number one represents the 500 milligrams of calcium and the two represents the 1,000 milligrams, which had been divided by 500. Unfortunately, this cannot be done with food labels, because they do not provide the amount of milligrams from phosphorus or calcium.

After reviewing Table 6.1, you may think that you can no longer enjoy meat, cola drinks, and processed foods if you want to maintain

			Calcium to Phosphorus Ratio
Food	Calcium	Phosphorus	(approximate)
Almonds, 1 ounce	73 mg	150 mg	1:2
Beef, 3 ounces, cooked	8 mg	135 mg	1:17
Black beans, 1 cup boiled	103 mg	282 mg	1:3
Bread, white or French, 1 slice	35 mg	30 mg	1:1
Bread, whole wheat, 1 slice	20 mg	74 mg	1:4
Broccoli, cooked, 1 cup	94 mg	100 mg	1:1
Cake donut, 1	11 mg	55 mg	1:5
Cheese, hard, 1 ounce	204 mg	146 mg	1:1
Chicken, light/dark meat, 3.5 ounces cooked	15 mg	195 mg	1:13
Cola beverage, diet and regular, 12 ounces	0 mg	44 to 70 mg	0:44–70
Cookie, chocolate sandwich, 1	10 mg	96 mg	1:10
Hazelnuts, 1 ounce	55 mg	92 mg	1:2
Kale, 1 cup cooked	94 mg	36 mg	1:0
Lamb, 3.5 ounces, cooked	8 mg	140 mg	1:18
Milk (any variety), 1 cup	300 mg	230 mg	1:1
Muffin, blueberry (from mix), 1	14 mg	80 mg	1:4
Peanuts, 1 ounce	15 mg	100 mg	1:7
Pinto beans, 1 cup boiled	82 mg	273 mg	1:3
Pork, 3.5 ounces, cooked	10 mg	200 mg	1:20
Potato chips, 1 ounce	7 mg	43 mg	1:6
Turkey, light/dark meat, 3.5 ounces	25 mg	214 mg	1:9
Turnip greens, boiled, 1 cup	198 mg	42 mg	1:0
Yogurt, 1 cup	400 mg	300 mg	1:1

TABLE 6.1. THE CALCIUM TO PHOSPHORUS RATIOS OF COMMON FOODS

a proper calcium balance. Fortunately, that's not true! Although too much phosphorus can upset the balance of calcium in the body, as can too much protein, you still can enjoy phosphorus-rich foods without upsetting your calcium balance. Just be moderate with your intake of animal protein and processed foods, eating them only occasionally, and begin to eat more foods that contain calcium and phosphorus in proper proportions.

Vitamin D–Calcium's Transport Vehicle

Vitamin D has one of the most important jobs relative to calcium nutrition. It is essential for proper calcium absorption through the intestinal wall. With a vitamin D deficiency, even when there's adequate dietary calcium, calcium absorption will be significantly hampered, leaving the body undersupplied with calcium by about half of the amount that might normally be absorbed. Vitamin D also helps to promote bone mineralization and assists in regulating the level of blood calcium by helping to promote calcium withdrawal from the blood and by stimulating the kidneys to retain calcium. However, vitamin D also functions in the body in ways unrelated to calcium. Researchers have recently learned that vitamin D is found in numerous other tissues, such as the brain and nervous system, immune cells, and some cancer cells. This recognition has led to suggestions that vitamin D may be involved in the functioning of the body's immune system and possibly in cancer prevention. Phosphorus is also needed to help make vitamin D available for bone mineralization.

Since early times, vitamin D has been known as the "sunshine" vitamin. This is because the body can manufacture vitamin D from a compound that it makes from cholesterol when the skin is exposed to the rays of the sun. To synthesize adequate vitamin D, about fifteen to twenty minutes of sun exposure two to three times a week are all that is usually needed. Because vitamin D is one of the few vitamins that is found in relatively few foods, for many people the sun is the best source. However, being housebound or living in a climate where sun exposure is limited may result in too little vitamin D production. Also, as we age, the body's ability to make vitamin D from sun exposure seems to decrease.

The richest food sources of vitamin D are milk and cereals that have had vitamin D added to them, oily fish like salmon or sardines, organ meats, and egg yolks. Most other foods contain very little, if any, vitamin D.

A vitamin D deficiency invariably reflects the interactions among calcium, vitamin D, and bone. This is because of the interdependent activities in which they are involved. Without adequate vitamin D, bone mineralization and the formation of hydroxyapatite, the hard bone mineral compound containing primarily calcium and phosphorus, are hindered or inhibited. When a child does not get enough vitamin D, he or she will develop the classic bone-deforming disease known as *rickets,* a disease where bones contain too little mineral. In adults, this condition is known as *osteomalacia* or adult rickets. In children with rickets, bones take on a classic bowed-leg appearance. This is because they are so weak that they bend when they have to support the child's weight. Their teeth develop abnormally, the enamel may be defective, and the jaw may be misshapen. In adults, osteomalacia occurs primarily in women. Their bones become soft, the spine bends, and the legs become bowed. Since milk is fortified with vitamin D, rickets has been practically eliminated in developed countries, although it still affects large numbers of children in less industrialized regions worldwide. In addition, infants who are breast fed or get little sun exposure may need vitamin D supplementaion. But check with your pediatrician before giving an infant vitamin D supplementation.

There is another side to vitamin D, however. Because vitamin D is readily stored in the body, large amounts of it are highly toxic. When excessive amounts of vitamin D are consumed, the body will absorb too much calcium, and a surplus will be released into the blood. Then, in a process known as *calcification,* the body will deposit the excess calcium into soft tissues, such as the kidneys or the arteries. The end result can be the formation of kidney stones, or in severe cases, hardening of the tissues themselves. Vitamin D toxicity also can stimulate bone dismantling, which results in weakened bones. Vitamin D toxicity usually occurs from taking a vitamin D supplement—and not from too much sunlight or food.

If you think you should be taking a vitamin D supplement, consult your health-care professional before actually doing so. Do not decide on your own to supplement without professional advice—particularly if you are pregnant or nursing, if you have health problems, or if you are taking any type of medication.

Vitamin K–A Recently Discovered Interaction

Vitamin K is the fourth and last fat-soluble vitamin to have been discovered. It is well known for its role in blood clotting and was originally called the Koagulation vitamin, from which the name vitamin K was derived. Scientists have learned that vitamin K is also needed by calcium in its bone-building activity. Vitamin K is integral to the production of a bone-related protein called osteocalcin or bone GLA-protein, which is produced by the osteoblasts, or bone-forming cells. In bone formation, osteocalcin allows calcium to bind to bone by being involved in the initial step of bone mineralization. Also, in an as yet poorly understood process, it may help to regulate the bone mineralization process. The level of osteocalcin in the blood is used in some clinical and research settings as an indicator of the amount of bone being formed or broken down in a given period of time. For example, osteocalcin concentrations are elevated with increased skeletal growth, such as in adolescents who are laying down significant amounts of bone. It also has been shown to be decreased in certain disease states when increased bone dismantling is occurring.

For most of us, getting adequate vitamin K is fairly easy. This is because our bodies have the ability to synthesize this vitamin from bacteria that reside in the colon. On average, about half of our vitamin K needs can be met from these vitamin K-making microbes. Also, vitamin K is widely found in foods like meats, milk, eggs, cereals, fruits, tea, liver, and typically in vitamin-mineral fortified foods. In fact, vitamin K is found in some of the same foods that provide calcium. Particularly rich sources of both vitamin K and calcium are kale, broccoli, turnip greens, many other green leafy vegetables, and other members of the cabbage family. Under normal circumstances, there is little danger of a deficiency or of getting a toxic amount of vitamin K. Typical multivitamin supplements usually provide recommended amounts of this vitamin. But, of course, food sources of vitamin K are always the best choice.

Calcium's Less Famous Team Members

Less often discussed, but no less important to the calcium team are magnesium, zinc, and fluoride. They interact with calcium in a variety of functions, some in bone health and some in the body's overall well-being. Interestingly, the best dietary sources of many of calcium's team members are foods that also contain calcium.

Magnesium

Since the days of the ancient Romans, magnesia alba—the white magnesium salts from the region of Magnesia in Greece from which magnesium was eventually named—have been touted for their many healing properties. Magnesium is probably most well known for its laxative properties as part of milk of magnesia or Epsom salts. However, it was not until the 1800s that magnesium was isolated chemically by the same scientist who had isolated calcium, Sir Humphry Davy. And it wasn't until the early 1900s that scientists were able to prove that magnesium was an essential mineral.

Magnesium's most familiar link to calcium is in its role as a component of the hardened mineral complex in the skeleton, hydroxyapatite, some of which can be made available, like calcium, to meet the body's needs. Magnesium also works closely with calcium in helping to regulate muscle activity, blood-clotting reactions, and blood-pressure regulation. Like calcium, when there is an inadequate amount of magnesium, it is also withdrawn from the skeleton. Magnesium also performs numerous essential functions in the body that are unrelated to calcium. It serves as part of more than 300 of the body's enzyme systems—special kinds of protein molecules that help regulate body functions—helps to produce energy, and is important in the production of proteins.

Reports of a severe magnesium deficiency are extremely rare. Effects are not apparent except when accompanied by disease. In fact, a magnesium deficiency is seen primarily in certain disease states, such as kidney disease, or in cases where the body doesn't have the ability to absorb magnesium. The effects develop slowly because magnesium stores in the blood can be called upon to meet the body's needs. A serious deficiency of magnesium is often accompanied by low blood calcium levels and causes a tetany similar to the calcium tetany described in Chapter 2. This is when muscles become unable to contract and relax properly, and they go into uncontrolled spasms. Other common symptoms include disorientation and confusion. Relative to the effects on calcium, less vitamin D is absorbed, because magnesium helps to mediate its transport through the intestinal wall. In turn, the calcium-vitamin D relationship is impacted, causing less calcium to be absorbed. Getting too much magnesium is also very uncommon, except in certain medical conditions, for example, where large amounts of magnesium are used therapeutically or when the ability to eliminate magnesium from the body is blunted. This is because the kidneys can eliminate large amounts of the mineral before they rise to dangerous levels.

Magnesium is fairly widespread in foods. The best food sources are unrefined and unprocessed plant foods, such as whole grains, nuts, and cooked dry beans. The milling or refining of grains, such as preparing white flour from whole-wheat flour or white rice from brown rice, results in most of the magnesium being discarded. Leafy, green vegetables are also good sources since magnesium is a component of the green pigment in plants, chlorophyll, which enables plants to transform carbon dioxide and water into carbohydrates. Hard water—the kind that leaves rings around the bathtub and around the teapot—is also rich in magnesium, as well as being high in calcium. When water is softened to eliminate the bathtub rings and mineral deposits in the teapot, magnesium and calcium are lost and are replaced by sodium.

Experts agree wholeheartedly that it is best to obtain magnesium from food. For the most part, supplementation with magnesium isn't considered necessary, and there is no conclusive evidence that the magnesium that is contained in calcium supplements is nutritionally superior to calcium supplements without magnesium. Always check with your health-care professional to see if supplements are right for you.

Zinc

Zinc's relationship with calcium, phosphorus, and magnesium is as an integral part of hydroxyapatite. Additionally, zinc is an indispensable partner in bone metabolism. Zinc also helps to form the collagen matrix on which calcium and other minerals are laid and may be involved with the activity of osteoblasts, the bone-forming cells. However, unlike calcium, much less zinc can be withdrawn from the skeletal reservoir if the body is in need.

Zinc was not recognized as an essential nutrient until the early 1960s. Now, we know that the body needs zinc for hundreds of vital functions unrelated to calcium or bone. Zinc is found in virtually every cell in the body. It is part of more than seventy different enzyme systems in the body. For example, zinc is necessary for growth and development, and is associated with the hormone insulin to help control blood sugar. It is also involved in the body's immune system and is needed for the production of proteins and genetic material.

Foods that provide the best sources of zinc are protein-rich foods such as meats, fish, poultry, liver, and shellfish—especially oysters. Cooked dry beans, peas, and lentils and whole grains are good sources, when large amounts are consumed. This is because zinc from plant foods is less well absorbed through the intestinal tract than are animal sources. In addition, unleavened grain products— those made without baking soda, baking powder, or yeast—like flat breads, contain phytic acid, also called phytates. Phytates are dietary constituents found in whole grains, legumes, and seeds, and are discussed in Chapter 7. Phytates bind with zinc (as well as with calcium) and prevent it from being absorbed. In leavened baked products, the phytates are broken down during the baking process, making zinc more available for absorption. The amount of useable zinc in vegetables varies widely, depending upon the zinc content of the soil in which they are grown.

Severe zinc deficiency was initially reported in the 1960s in Middle Eastern children and adolescent males who were suffering from severe growth retardation and stunted sexual development. In the bones, a zinc deficiency causes a defect in collagen development, thereby reducing calcium's activity in bone mineralization. As a result, the lack of zinc causes abnormal bone growth, and bone cell activity is impacted.

A severe zinc deficiency is generally uncommon in Western countries, but some groups, such as older postmenopausal women are known to take in too little zinc. New research suggests that a high calcium intake, especially accompanied by an inadequate zinc intake, may increase the potential for a zinc deficiency. Increasing zinc intake should go hand in hand with increasing calcium. However, these findings don't mean that you should automatically be taking a zinc supplement, but it underscores the importance of insuring an adequate and balanced intake of nutrients in general. If you choose to supplement, women should limit the amount to 12 mg per day and men to 15 mg per day, which are the current recommendations for adults. Some calcium supplements come with zinc added to them, but if you already take a multivitamin-mineral supplement that contains zinc or if you eat a vitamin-mineral fortified breakfast cereal, you do not need to take such a supplement. In amounts just slightly higher than recommended and taken on a regular basis, zinc has been shown to affect cholesterol levels and may hasten the development of heart disease. Thus, in this case, a little more may not be better. Getting too much zinc also can impair the immune system and may also impact the absorption of copper, another mineral that is needed by the body.

Fluoride

Although fluoride is widely dispersed in the body's tissues, the body contains only a trace amount, especially relative to the amount of calcium, phosphorus, magnesium, and zinc. Fluoride's relationship with calcium is as a component of the calcium-phosphorus crystals of hydroxyapatite, which forms a very hard compound called fluoroapatite. Fluoroapatite helps strengthen the bones and increases the teeth's resistance to cavities by making them more resistant to bacterial-acid production that leads to dental caries. In fact, the decline in cavities over the past forty years in developed countries has been attributed to the widespread use of fluoride. In addition, a few early studies have suggested that fluoride may offer some protection from osteoporosis by helping to strengthen bones.

Nearly all typical human diets contain some fluoride, although the amount in plant foods and animal products is largely dependent on the soil, water, or amount in the feed. The richest natural sources are fish with edible bones such as canned salmon and most tea leaves. The most reliable and significant source of fluoride is fluoridated drinking water. Fluoridation of water came about from scientific observations in the 1930s, which suggested that naturally fluoridated water at the proper concentrations reduced dental caries. Currently, about one-half of the United States population has access to fluoridated water. Fluoridated toothpastes and other dental products are also reliable sources of this element.

A fluoride deficiency appears to be relatively uncommon in well-nourished, industrialized populations. Very little is needed to benefit from its protective effect. Although a shortage of fluoride results in weakened tooth enamel and increased susceptibility to tooth decay, there do not appear to be any known metabolic effects from a lack of fluoride.

Excess fluoride, during tooth enamel formation, causes blotchy, discolored teeth with brown stains, a condition called *fluorosis* or *teeth mottling*. Too much fluoride also has been shown to cause the bones to lose their natural color and luster, to become soft and porous, and to be more easily fractured. However, under normal conditions, there is little concern about the average person getting too much fluoride from dietary sources, dental products, or fluoridated drinking water. The exception is small children who may swallow an excessive amount of fluoridated toothpaste or other fluoridated dental products. Thus, supervision of children during teeth brushing when fluoridated products are used is strongly recommended. Other problems with fluoride toxicity have been limited to rare situations where a public water system had failed and fluoride concentrations became excessively high.

Vitamin C

Vitamin C, or ascorbic acid, has been appreciated for centuries for preventing scurvy, the historically devastating cause of suffering and death in sailors. Scurvy, among other things, causes loose teeth, bleeding and rotting gums, impaired wound healing, and muscle weakness. Vitamin C is also well known for its highly touted, although scientifically unproven, role in preventing and curing the common cold. But among its established functions in the body, vitamin C is needed for the formation of collagen, the cornerstone compound of the fibrous network on which calcium and other bone-related minerals are laid down. Without enough vitamin C, the formation of the bones' collagen network is hampered. After several weeks on a diet lacking in vitamin C, bone building falters to the point that the body's long bones, like the leg bone, become softened, painful, and deformed. Fractures can appear and the teeth become loose. There also is evidence that vitamin C may even help calcium be absorbed from the intestinal tract.

By far, citrus fruits are among the best sources of vitamin C, with the kiwi fruit being among the richest sources. Strawberries, dark leafy greens, cabbage, broccoli, tomatoes, and peppers are also excellent sources of this vitamin, some of which are also high in calcium (like kale and broccoli). Milk and other animal foods, except liver, are poor sources of vitamin C.

Generally, most healthy people easily get more than the recommended amount of vitamin C, which is 60 milligrams for adults. Three-fourths of a cup of orange juice has 75 milligrams. By far, we get much more than the small amount needed to prevent scurvy, which is only 10 milligrams a day. However, those with special health problems such as heavy metal poisoning and those who are suffering from extensive burns require significantly higher amounts of vitamin C. Furthermore, people who smoke have higher needs and should get at least 100 milligrams of vitamin C per day.

Nutrition experts agree that it is best to get vitamin C from food. However, if you choose to supplement with vitamin C, your body will excrete any excess in your urine. For adults, 1,000 to 2,000 milligrams of vitamin C per day should not pose a great risk of toxicity. However, people taking more than 2,000 milligrams per day have experienced nausea, diarrhea, abdominal cramps, kidney stones, and even loss of bone mineral. Note, too, that large doses of this vitamin may obscure the results of medical tests used to detect diabetes and are dangerous for people with iron overload. Check with your health-care professional before supplementing with vitamin C.

Vitamin A

In addition to its role in night vision, vitamin A also is involved in body functions such as maintaining healthy skin, developing healthy bones and teeth, and helping to support a robust immune system. Vitamin A interacts with calcium, primarily in the bone-mineralization process. The proper amount of vitamin A is needed for the manufacture of the collagen matrix on which calcium is deposited. A vitamin A deficiency impairs calcium's ability to form strong bones and results in a skeleton that contains too little mineral. Excessive amounts of vitamin A have been found to increase the amount of calcium in the blood, which disrupts blood calcium balance. Vitamin A toxicity most often occurs from supplement abuse and is unlikely to occur from dietary intake. This vitamin is stored in the liver where it can potentially build up to toxic levels. In the average healthy person, it can take as long as two years to become vitamin A depleted. Vitamin A toxicity, called *hypervitaminosis A,* affects nearly all body systems. Consequences include headaches, vomiting, cracked and peeling skin, bone and joint pain, blindness, and impaired functioning of the immune system.

We get vitamin A in two ways: from plants and from animals. From plants, vitamin A comes from precursor compounds called carotenoids, like beta-carotene, which are converted by the body to the active form of vitamin A. Carotenoids are abundant in deep yellow and orange-fleshed fruits and vegetables like peaches, apricots, carrots, sweet potatoes, and winter squash, and dark leafy greens like spinach, broccoli, kale, and turnip greens. It is impossible to get a toxic amount of vitamin A from plant foods regardless of how much is consumed.

In animal foods, we get the active form of vitamin A directly. Fortified milk, butter, eggs, and liver are among the best sources. When you depend on a balanced diet for your nutrients, it is unlikely that you would get too much vitamin A. However, excessive consumption of liver has been associated with vitamin A toxicity.

Supplementing with vitamin A is not recommended. This is specifically true for pregnant women, because vitamin A is known to cause birth defects. Check with your health-care professional before supplementing with this vitamin.

Dietary Fiber—Calcium's Friend or Foe?

Dietary fiber is the part of a plant that the body cannot break down during normal digestion. Essentially, fiber travels though the intestinal tract without being absorbed into the bloodstream. When most fiber reaches the colon, it is in more or less the same form as it was when it was eaten. Fiber is found only in plant foods that have not been refined or milled. There's some fiber in all fruits, vegetables, whole grains, cooked dry beans, peas, lentils, nuts, and seeds. Refined grain foods like white rice or those made from white flour contain virtually no fiber, and there is never any fiber in animal foods like meat, milk, and eggs. Fiber-rich foods are also abundant in protective phytochemicals (*phyto* means plant), many of which are lost during refining. Phytochemicals, such as flavonoids, carotenoids, and tocopherols, which possess antioxidant activity that helps to prevent cell damage, and numerous other compounds that interfere with cancer growth are among the numerous substances found only in plant foods. Many high-fiber foods also contain some calcium. These include broccoli, dried figs, cooked dry beans, almonds, and hazelnuts.

Fiber plays a major role in proper bowel function and easy elimination, and evidence suggests that it may also help to protect against colon cancer, diverticular disease, diabetes, and heart disease. Despite the health benefits of eating a high fiber diet, there is considerable debate over whether or not fiber interferes with calcium absorption. However, many people are unaware that there are many distinct kinds of fiber, and that the different types of fiber act differently in the body.

Types of Fiber

Dietary fiber is usually classified into two main groups according to their solubility in water: Fibers that hold on to fluid in the intestine are called insoluble fiber; other fibers, called soluble fiber, become gel-like and gummy, and do not hold on to water. The most common types of insoluble fibers are cellulose, many hemicelluloses, and lignins, while the soluble fibers also include some kinds of hemicelluloses, and also gums, pectins, and mucilages. Foods nearly always contain a mixture of both insoluble and soluble fiber, but are usually identified as being abundant in one kind. For example, oats are known for being rich in soluble fiber, while whole wheat is recognized for its abundance of insoluble fiber.

Often called "nature's broom," insoluble fibers essentially sweep the undigested matter from food through the intestinal tract. They add bulk and softness to the stools and promote regularity of bowel movements. Also, a diet high in insoluble fiber has been linked to a reduced risk of colon cancer. Foods high in insoluble fiber are whole wheat breads and pastas, brown rice, corn, and popcorn. Insoluble fiber is also abundant in the edible skin of fruits, potatoes, carrots, and many other root vegetables.

Foods high in soluble fiber include oats, barley, cooked dry beans, peas, lentils, several fruits such as apples and citrus fruits, and vegetables such as carrots. The soluble fiber in these foods becomes gummy and thick and binds to fat-related substances, like bile acids or cholesterol, and helps them pass through the intestines as waste. Soluble fiber also lengthens the time it takes for food to travel through the digestive tract, which helps slow the absorption of sugar—a benefit for people with diabetes or those who have trouble keeping their blood sugar in control. Soluble fiber may also foster weight control. This may be because high fiber foods provide bulk to the diet and leave the stomach more slowly, extending the feeling of fullness or satisfaction after a meal.

High Fiber Diets and Calcium Absorption

Fiber's effect on calcium absorption is determined by the type and the amount of dietary fiber consumed and by how much calcium you are getting. Generally, the fiber contained in fruits and vegetables has little effect on calcium absorption, while the fiber found in whole grains has a somewhat greater effect. A few studies have found that an extremely high intake of a specific kind of insoluble fiber, cellulose, which is particularly abundant in wheat bran, blocks some calcium absorption.

Some short-term studies, many of which have been only a few weeks or so in duration, have demonstrated that a very high fiber intake of about 100 grams per day may have a significant impact on calcium absorption. However, it has been found that in people who consume a balanced high-fiber diet with adequate calcium, fiber does not appear to interfere with calcium absorption. Some experts believe that this is due to the body's potential to adapt to a high-fiber intake by increasing the amount of calcium it absorbs—similar to the changes in calcium absorption that occur at different stages of life, which are discussed in Chapter 7.

Most of the impact on calcium absorption from consumption of high-fiber diets may occur because of phytic acid and oxalic acid—which are dietary constituents found in plant foods. Neither of these

compounds is classed as a fiber, but both are often mistakenly identified as fiber. This is because both are naturally found in fiber-
containing foods. Phytic acid is abundant in the outer husks of
whole grains, legumes, and seeds. Oxalic acid is found in only a few
foods such as spinach, Swiss chard, beet greens, collard greens, and
rhubarb. Both phytic acid and oxalic acid bind with calcium in the
intestines, which is then lost from the body with other wastes. However, in the case of oxalic acid, only the calcium contained in the
food itself is lost. Absorption of the additional calcium in other
foods eaten along with the oxalic acid-rich food is not affected. It is
thought that the typical amounts of phytic acid and oxalic acid that
are consumed by Americans is not sufficient to seriously affect overall calcium absorption. (See Chapter 7 for additional information
concerning phytic and oxalic acid.) But if this is of concern to you,
try cooking or serving phytic- and oxalic-rich foods with lemon
juice, lime juice, or vinegar. The acid in these foods will help release
some of the calcium for absorption.

Adapting to a High-Fiber Diet with Calcium

People who consume a typical animal-based Western diet average
about only 10 to 12 grams of fiber per day in contrast to the 20 to 30
grams that are recommended. However, the human body does not
adapt instantly to increases in fiber intake, so there may be some
temporary side effects. The most common and most complained
about side effect, though not serious, is bloating and flatulence, or
intestinal gas. This is due to bacteria in the colon that ferment the
fiber and produce gas as part of their digestive waste products. The
most serious effect, which rarely occurs, is intestinal blockage or impacted stools. This results from increasing fiber too fast and not
drinking enough fluids while increasing fiber intake. Because fiber
absorbs water, fluid intake along with fiber intake must be increased
at the same time. Another temporary effect of increasing fiber intake

is that there may be a small increase in calcium loss. Whether this is due to the fiber itself or the phytic or oxalic acids in fiber-rich foods is a matter that needs further research. After a few weeks of gradually adding fiber to your diet, most people adapt and these effects subside.

Basically, the answer to fiber and calcium intake is simple: For the amount of fiber that the typical American consumes, there's little concern about a significant negative effect on calcium absorption. By far, it's advisable to increase your fiber intake as well as your calcium intake. You can take a major step to improve the typical low intake of both fiber and calcium by eating more calcium-rich plant foods and by replacing processed food products with unrefined foods. The potential benefits are substantial.

Protein—The Great Calcium Thief

Coined by the Greeks as meaning "of first importance," protein, which is found in both plant and animal foods, is essential to our bodies for growth and proper development. In fact, we cannot live without this essential nutrient. The building blocks of protein are known as amino acids, of which there are twenty of importance in human nutrition. For the most part, our bodies function properly whether we get amino acids from animal foods or from a mixture of plant foods. However, the amino acids that are more abundant in animal proteins can affect the retention of calcium by the body differently than the kind of amino acids found in plant foods.

Animal protein—like that found in steak or chicken—is the traditional "centerpiece" of the typical Western meal. This main course is essentially calcium-free. The bones, of course, contain calcium, but unlike other meat-eating animals, we don't eat the bones along with the meat. To get around this, we could boil the meat bones in vinegar, which would cause them to soften and release their calcium into the liquid. A few groups of people actually do this as part of the preparation of traditional soups or stews, but it is uncommon. Whether it is beef, veal, lamb, pork, fish, eggs, or poultry, a high intake of animal protein can adversely affect calcium nutrition.

Protein's Effects on Calcium

The potential effects of protein on the body's calcium status depend largely on the kind of protein and how much protein we consume. The typical high intake of animal proteins creates an environment in the body that causes an increased excretion of this mineral in the urine. One of the digestive products of protein is sulfuric acid, which is higher in animal proteins than plant proteins. Sulfuric acid increases the acidity of the urine. To help lower the urine's acidity, calcium, as one of the body's main buffers—that is, acid neutralizers—is drawn from the blood. Consequently, it is eliminated through the urine when sulfuric acid is eliminated by the kidneys. When there is inadequate dietary calcium to replenish calcium loss, calcium is withdrawn from the skeleton.

When protein intake is within the recommended daily amounts of 0.75 to 0.80 grams of protein per kilogram of body weight (2.2 pounds equals a kilogram) or between 50 and 60 grams per day for average healthy adults, the amount of calcium that is excreted in the urine is about the amount that normally occurs in an average healthy person. On the other hand, the more protein we consume, the more calcium we lose. For example, doubling protein intake can lead to about a 50 percent increase in calcium excretion. Further, over a prolonged period of time, if these calcium losses are accompanied by a calcium-deficient diet and thus are not replaced, bones may become weakened.

Plant proteins produce less sulfuric acid in the digestive process and thus produce a less acidic urine. Groups of people who rely on plant-based proteins from legumes, such as cooked dry beans, peas, lentils, grains, seeds, and nuts, tend to experience less urinary calcium loss than those whose diets center around animal foods. They also tend to eat less protein in general, and so, from the start, their calcium stores are at less risk.

Protein and Bone Health

International comparisons of hip fracture rates show that as protein intake increases, so do hip fracture rates. In non-industrialized regions, such as Africa and in some parts of Asia, where plant foods are the primary sources of protein, hip fractures are rare. In contrast, in Northern European countries and in the United States, where animal-based proteins are the mainstay, rates of hip fractures are significantly higher.

The Protein Overdose

Consuming about 75 grams of protein each day is sufficient to cause enough calcium excretion from the body to prompt the removal of calcium from the skeleton—potentially leading to a chronic loss of calcium from the bones over time. To put this into perspective, protein intake can easily add up to 75 grams in an animal-based diet.

Consider this example: The diet analysis report of one student showed that he had eaten 95 grams of protein in one day. His diet for that day included the following: for breakfast he had two fried eggs, a sausage patty, and buttered toast, totaling about 22 grams of protein; for lunch he had two cheeseburger patties on a bun, fries, a milkshake, and coleslaw, totaling about 44 grams of protein; and for dinner he had about 6 ounces of broiled chicken, white rice, and steamed green beans, totaling about 35 grams of protein.

Does this menu sound extreme? It really isn't. Government studies have shown that the average man eats at least one 6-ounce serving of meat, fish, or poultry at each meal, and the average woman eats about one 3- to 4-ounce serving of meat, fish, or poultry at each meal. To illustrate the size of these portions, a 3- to 3½-ounce serving of cooked meat, fish, or poultry is about the size of a deck of playing cards. With about 7 grams of protein per ounce of meat, fish, or poultry, it is readily apparent how easily the amount of animal protein can add up.

The potential negative effects on calcium from a high animal protein diet does not necessitate eliminating meat from your diet, although nutritionists would agree that eating more plant food and less animal food is healthier. There are a few strategies that will help you lessen the potential long-term losses of calcium due to excess protein consumption. Try to slowly and moderately switch from having animal food as the "centerpiece" of your meals to centering your meals around plant foods. Gradually work up to this by thinking first of pasta, rice, beans, lentils, split peas, and tofu as the foods around which you plan your meal. Start by making small changes, which are known to significantly help guarantee success. For example, one day per week increase the serving size of rice, pasta, bread, or potatoes, while slightly decreasing the portion of meat. Particularly in stews, casseroles, and other mixed dishes, a smaller amount of meat usually goes unnoticed, and the extra pasta or rice helps to make the meal satisfying. Over time, advance to making at least one meal per week entirely plant-based. There are thousands of hearty plant-based recipes, some of which are likely to please almost any size appetite and palate. Ideas for cookbooks and sources that include calcium-rich, plant-based recipes can be found in the Additional Resources at the end of this book.

Over time, you will come to enjoy these changes, and they will become a part of your regular diet. And not only will you reap the health benefits of plant-based eating, but the economic benefits as well. One of the less-touted benefits of plant-based eating is that it's less expensive than an animal-based diet.

Getting the Proper Proportion

If the plant-based approach lacks appeal, try basing your food choices according to the ratio of calcium to protein. It has been suggested that a beneficial ratio of calcium to protein is 16:1 or more. This means that you should get at least 16 milligrams of calcium for every 1 gram of animal-based protein that you consume. Unfortunately, it is much more common to get more protein than calcium. For example, the average American consumes a calcium to protein ratio of about 9:1. Compare the foods listed in Table 6.2 below. Where do you make most of your choices?

TABLE 6.2. CALCIUM TO PROTEIN RATIO OF SELECTED ANIMAL-BASED FOODS	
Animal Protein Sources	**Calcium to Protein Ratio** (grams of calcium to protein)
Beef, pork, lamb, and veal, 3 ounces	3:1
Cheese, 1 ounce	30:1
Cheese, Ricotta, 1 cup	24:1
Chicken or turkey, 3 ounces	2:1
Milk, 1 cup	38:1
Salmon (canned, with bones), 3 ounces	12:1
Sardines (canned, with bones), 3 ounces	15:1
Seafood, 3 ounces	2:1
Yogurt, 1 cup	44:1

Some Final Words

Calcium is undeniably indispensable for health and well-being, but its ability to perform its functions is often dependent on other compounds, like vitamin D, and vice versa. Some of the most central roles of calcium in bone metabolism are at the crossroads of where many interactions between calcium and other nutrients occur. These interdependencies are so important that if our dietary calcium intake is inadequate, if we don't absorb enough calcium through the intestinal tract, or if we excrete too much calcium through the kidneys, the body's functioning is affected. The significance of an ample intake of calcium each day cannot be overemphasized.

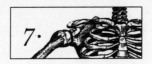

7.

Factors in Calcium Absorption

THE HUMAN body is a remarkable machine, beautifully orches-
trated to ensure that we get the most benefit from the foods we eat.
But first, the body must change the food we eat into useable forms.
Until these dietary constituents pass through the walls of the intestines, what we have eaten is still "outside" the body and is of little use to us. For example, when we eat an almond, the digestive
system breaks it down into its smallest parts, but those parts—including protein, calcium, phytochemicals, and fibers—are still outside of the body. They must be absorbed into the body in order for
the body to benefit.

The calcium in the almond, like all other minerals and vitamins,
is not broken down into smaller components. The body essentially
absorbs it in the same form in which it existed in the almond. But
for the calcium to be absorbed, the environment in the intestinal
tract must be right. Dietary constituents found along with calcium in
food and the state of the body are deciding factors in how much calcium, if any at all, will be carried across the intestinal wall.

Getting Calcium into the Body

To be absorbed, calcium must be "freed" from the ingested food. This occurs during the digestive process. Digestion is the process of breaking down food into smaller components that the body can absorb. It starts in the mouth with the mechanical breakdown of the food by chewing, which results in smaller particles that travel down the esophagus—a tube that goes from the mouth to the stomach. More digestion occurs in the stomach and is completed in the small intestine. The small intestine is where the majority of calcium, other nutrients, phytochemicals, and other dietary constituents are absorbed into the bloodstream for delivery to all parts of the body.

Factors That Promote Calcium Absorption

Several factors enhance calcium absorption. The amount of calcium that makes it through the intestinal wall depends largely on the stage of life, the environment in the intestinal tract, the food sources of calcium, and the mixture of foods being consumed.

Times of Growth When the body is growing and developing, calcium needs are increased. During pregnancy, breastfeeding, childhood, and adolescence, the amount of calcium that is absorbed by the body is much higher than it is at other times during life. Women who are pregnant or breastfeeding, infants, children, and adolescents during their growth spurts absorb at least half of their dietary calcium; that is, the calcium they consume. Infants can absorb up to three-fourths of their calcium intake, while normal adults—who aren't growing—absorb a little less than a third of the calcium they consume.

An Acidic Stomach Environment After the first bite of food, or sometimes even when we are thinking about eating—especially a mouth-watering and appetizing food—special hormones are signaled by the brain to begin secreting gastric acid into the stomach. Gastric acid, also called stomach acid, produces an acidic environment in the stomach. It functions to kill and prevent growth of harmful bacteria that enter the body with foods and contributes to some protein digestion. An acidic environment also enhances absorption of calcium in the upper portion of the small intestine where the digestive contents are still somewhat acidic after leaving the stomach.

For most of our lives, the stomach secretes the proper amount of gastric acid. But, generally, as we get older, less stomach acid is produced. In turn, less calcium gets absorbed. So, insuring ample daily calcium intake and choosing foods that are especially good sources becomes even more important as we age.

Presence of Lactose Since 1926, we have known that milk sugar, or lactose, a natural component of dairy foods, helps calcium be absorbed, especially in infants. As you will learn in Chapter 9, many adults aren't able to tolerate lactose. Fortunately, a deficiency or lack of lactose doesn't appear to severely disable the body's ability to absorb calcium when a normal diet is consumed. (See Chapter 9 for information about lactose intolerance.)

Adequate Vitamin D As you learned in Chapter 6, vitamin D and calcium are inextricably linked. This is because vitamin D plays several important roles in calcium nutrition. Indeed, this vitamin is essential to calcium absorption. It stimulates the production of a specific protein called calbindin, which is responsible for intestinal absorption of calcium, and also causes some cellular changes in the intestinal wall that facilitate calcium transport. Without vitamin D, calcium absorption is severely hampered.

Consuming Calcium and Phosphorus in About the Same Amounts Scientists have long believed that intestinal transport of calcium is helped when dietary calcium and phosphorus are consumed together in about the same amounts. As you learned in Chapter 6, relying too much on processed foods and cola beverages may result in a calcium–phosphorus imbalance. When there is too much or too little phosphorus present, calcium can be lost from the body before it gets absorbed.

Factors That Interfere with Calcium Absorption

Interactions among calcium and other dietary constituents that inhibit its activities are not limited to functions within the body. The sheer process of calcium absorption is complex. There are several things that can interfere with calcium's transport through the intestinal wall. However, these generally are attributed to dietary excesses, which can compete with calcium for absorption. When dietary intake is balanced, problems with calcium absorption are usually of little concern.

Dietary Fat On a regular basis, eating too much fat of any kind is not good for anyone's general health. Saturated fats, though—the kind that are found primarily in animal foods and are linked with heart disease—can combine with calcium and form compounds called soaps, which prevent calcium from being absorbed. Calcium is then eliminated from the body along with the soaps. Since saturated fats tend to be high in protein-rich, animal-based diets, calcium may be subject to double jeopardy—that is, it is vulnerable to being lost before it is absorbed and at risk for increased loss through the urine due to the effects of protein metabolism (see Chapter 6). Other types of fat, such as those found in vegetables, nuts, and seeds do not appear to affect calcium absorption, except in certain medical conditions, such as steatorrhea, where the body is unable to absorb fat.

In this case, these types of fats also form soaps, preventing calcium from being absorbed. In addition, a particular non-food based oil, mineral oil, also prevents calcium from being absorbed in the same manner as other fats. Mineral oil is a petroleum-based product that has been used as a fat substitute and is still used by many people as a laxative. Not only does it prevent calcium from being absorbed, but it also has the same effect on phosphorus, carotenoids, and vitamins A, D, and K—all of which in some way interact with calcium.

Cellulose Cellulose is one of several different components that are collectively known as dietary fiber. Fiber is a general term for the indigestible portions of plants—specifically the bran or husk of a grain kernel and the skins and seeds of fruits and vegetables; there is no fiber in animal foods. Most types of dietary fibers have little or no effect on calcium absorption.

However, large amounts of cellulose, particularly accompanied by an imbalanced, low-calcium diet, have been found to interfere with absorption of some calcium. At this time, though, further studies are needed to conclude whether or not there are long-term consequences. Cellulose is found in abundance especially in wheat bran, a concentrated source of fiber that is popular for increasing fiber intake. If you are concerned about your fiber intake, the message here is that it is best to consume a wide variety of fiber-rich foods rather than relying on one isolated source. (For more information on fiber and calcium, see Chapter 6.)

Alcohol Consumption of a moderate amount of alcohol has been associated with positive health effects such as protection against heart disease. However, chronically imbibing more than a moderate amount of alcohol has negative effects on calcium absorption. Regardless of the kind of alcoholic beverage—wine, beer, or hard liquor—an excessive amount disrupts the absorption process by its indirect effects on vitamin D metabolism. With too much alcohol too often, the liver becomes less efficient at activating vitamin D. Thus, calcium is excreted before it can be utilized.

Caffeine The predominant sources of caffeine for Americans are coffee, espresso, tea, cocoa, and carbonated beverages. Several studies have documented that caffeine creates a climate in the body that causes calcium to be excreted from the intestinal tract and lost in the feces. But this effect appears to be of concern primarily in people with calcium-deficient diets who consume large amounts of caffeine-containing beverages. A daily intake equivalent to one to two cups of coffee coupled with a proper dietary calcium intake or the amount of milk typically added to a café latte usually offsets the amount of calcium that is lost in healthy people.

Sodium Salt, or table salt—about 40 percent of which is sodium— has been esteemed since antiquity. The ancient Greeks and Romans valued it so highly that it was used to pay their soldiers. In fact, the word salary is derived from the Latin term for salt money. In the present times, though, salt and sodium have become highly valued constituents of the American diet—which contains notoriously high amounts of them. Large amounts of sodium are hidden in processed and convenience foods and fast foods, and many people liberally use the salt shaker at the table. Even most unrefined, un-processed foods contain some sodium, but not enough to be of concern. Too much dietary sodium causes calcium to be lost in the urine before the body can use it. The long-term concern is a potential increased risk of osteoporosis if more calcium is withdrawn from the bones than replaced. Moderate salt and sodium intake is advised.

Oxalic Acid Calcium in some plant foods is complexed with a compound called oxalic acid, which makes the calcium virtually un-absorbable. Calcium oxalates are abundant in vegetables, such as spinach, Swiss chard, beet greens, collard greens, and rhubarb. Chocolate even contains a small amount of calcium oxalate. For example, only 5 percent of the calcium from spinach can be absorbed, because the rest is bound to oxalic acid. Although the calcium in these particular foods is unavailable, don't eliminate them from your diet. They are packed with other nutrients and phytochemicals that compensate for the unavailable calcium. Also, keep in mind that these aren't the typical or most common foods from which we obtain calcium.

Moreover, the amount of calcium that is prevented from being absorbed because of the calcium oxalate complex is limited to the calcium contained in the food itself. Additional calcium contained in other foods consumed at the same time retain their normal degree of absorbability. At the current intake level of oxalic acid in American diets, calcium oxalates are not considered to be a significant problem.

Phytic acid Phytic acid is a dietary constituent that is found in the outer layers of legumes, seeds, unrefined grains, such as whole wheat and barley, and in unleavened grain products, like Middle Eastern-style flat breads. It is well known that in unleavened products and as it occurs naturally in whole grains, legumes, and seeds, phytic acid binds with calcium and prevents its absorption through the intestinal tract. However, when leavening agents, such as yeast, baking powder, or baking soda are used in grain products, phytic acid is inactivated and no longer affects mineral absorption. At the current intake levels of phytic acid by Americans, phytic acid's effect on calcium absorption is not thought to be of significance. Also, studies have suggested that the body may adapt to higher intakes and that the effects on calcium absorption may balance out over time. Moreover, in the emerging science of phytochemicals, it appears that phytic acid may be protective against some types of cancer.

Medication Use When we take medication, prescription or over-the-counter, there are often potential interactions with calcium and other nutrients. As you learned in Chapter 3, there are numerous medications that may interact with calcium. Some can reduce the amount of calcium that gets absorbed through the intestinal wall, while others can interfere with calcium's work inside the body (see Table 3.1 on page 16). When receiving or filling a prescription, be sure to ask your health-care professional or pharmacist about any known medication-nutrient interactions and what you should do about them.

Some Final Words

Calcium from food will not be useful and won't provide any benefits if it doesn't get through the intestinal wall and into the bloodstream. The body's ability to absorb calcium through the intestinal wall is the result of millions of years of evolution and normally works very well. Calcium absorption can vary greatly among individuals and under different conditions. In particular, as we think about the factors that promote or interfere with calcium absorption, balance and moderation in all things, including calcium, works in its favor.

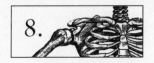

Getting Calcium in the
Right Amounts

To SUPPORT calcium needs and replace normal losses, we require a relatively large amount of this essential nutrient everyday throughout our entire lives. But most Americans do not get enough calcium, and this is true for just about every age, gender, and ethnic group. Even more alarming is that no single group of women—at nearly any stage of life—consumes enough calcium to meet the current recommendations.

In general, women of childbearing age get only about two-thirds of their recommended calcium. Pregnant women, unless taking a calcium-containing prenatal supplement, on average get about only half of what they need. Moreover, postmenopausal women, who are at increased risk for bone loss and osteoporosis, consume less than half their calcium requirements.

In elderly men and women, the fastest growing group in the United States, current calcium intakes are inadequate to prevent calcium-related bone loss. (See Figure 8.1 on page 90, which compares the need for calcium at different stages of life versus actual

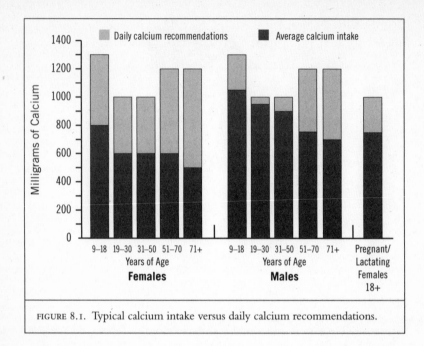

FIGURE 8.1. Typical calcium intake versus daily calcium recommendations.

intake.) Although not shown in the table, it appears that only young children are meeting their needs for calcium. However, we are seeing an increasing and alarming trend: Recent surveys show that boys and girls are decreasing their calcium intake, especially from milk, in favor of cola beverages, juices, and other calcium-poor beverages.

Dietary Recommendations for Calcium

Since most of the body's calcium is stockpiled in the bones, the recommendations for calcium intake have been determined largely by requirements to optimize skeletal health. Calcium needs vary by gender and stage of life. For women, factors like pregnancy, lactation, and menopause influence their needs.

Dietary recommendations for nutrients related to bone have been a high profile topic in recent years. The Food and Nutrition

Board of the National Research Council, an independent governmental body, has updated intake recommendations for calcium, as well as the other bone-related nutrients—phosphorus, magnesium, vitamin D, and fluoride. These recommendations are now found in the new Dietary Reference Intakes (DRIs). The DRIs replace our country's traditional fifty-year history with the Recommended Dietary Allowances (RDAs) and reflect our increased understanding of nutrient requirements and their unique roles in maintaining health.

The DRIs consist of four different kinds of nutrient recommendations that are designed for planning and evaluating diets of healthy people in the United States. They include average daily recommendations that are considered to be adequate to meet the known nutrient needs of most healthy people, as well as recommendations for the highest level of intake that appears safe. They are based on the latest scientific information for each stage of life, taking into consideration the roles of nutrients in helping to protect against major chronic diseases, such as osteoporosis. This is a departure from the traditional RDAs, which were based on preventing classic deficiency diseases like rickets and scurvy.

In 1998, the National Research Council proposed new gender and age-specific recommendations for calcium, as well as for phosphorus, magnesium, vitamin D, and fluoride. These are based on the latest scientific knowledge reflecting the amounts of these nutrients that are needed to maximize calcium retention by the body. Compared to the last RDAs, in general, calcium recommendations have been increased. The adult DRI for calcium ranges from 1,000 to 1,300 milligrams per day. The RDAs previously had ranged from 800 to 1,000 milligrams per day. This is in stark contrast to the average American's intake of 500 to 800 milligrams of calcium per day. See Table 8.1 on page 92 for a listing of calcium per age group and category. The following is a discussion of these recommendations.

TABLE 8.1. DIETARY REFERENCE INTAKES OF CALCIUM OVER THE LIFECYCLE		
Category	Age	Calcium Requirements
Infants	0 to 5 months:	210 mg
	6 to 11 months:	270 mg
Children and adolescents	1 to 3 years:	500 mg
	4 to 8 years:	800 mg
	9 to 18 years:	1,300 mg
Men	19 to 50 years:	1,000 mg
	over 50 years:	1,200 mg
Women, general	19 to 50 years:	1,000 mg
	over 50 years:	1,200 mg
Pregnant and breastfeeding females	up to 18 years:	1,300 mg
	19 to 50 years:	1,000 mg

Calcium Recommendations for Adults

Until sometime between the third and fourth decades of life, in most healthy adult men and women, bone remodeling occurs at about equal rates, with little bone loss resulting. During this part of the lifecycle, men and women normally lose only about one-half to one percent of bone each year. There are special situations, however, such as certain disease states or unhealthy lifestyles when bone loss may be accelerated.

Calcium intake recommendations during the adult years are based on the need to help maintain bone mass and to help prevent future bone fractures. Although men experience fewer bone fractures than women, studies have shown that the risk of breaking a bone increases in men who do not consume adequate calcium.

The new DRIs recommend that, until fifty years of age, adults of both sexes maintain a daily calcium intake of 1,000 milligrams— rather than the 800 milligrams recommended previously.

Calcium Recommendations for Pregnant and Breastfeeding Females

Ask any woman who has given birth, regardless of her understanding of physiology, and she will tell you without hesitation that significant changes take place in her body during pregnancy—not the least of which is the substantial stress that will be placed on her calcium stores. Not only does she need calcium to protect her bones, but she also needs to provide her unborn child with the calcium it needs for bone development and its own metabolism. Fortunately, when a pregnant woman maintains an adequate intake of calcium, there is no permanent decline in her own calcium stores. However, women who have low intakes of calcium during breastfeeding may lose significant amounts of calcium from their bones, due to the body's increased need for calcium in the production of breast milk.

The 1998 calcium recommendation for a pregnant woman between nineteen and fifty years old is 1,000 milligrams of calcium per day, which is the same as the recommendations for adults. However, for the pregnant female who is younger than eighteen years old and is still working on building her own bones, the recommendation is 1,300 milligrams per day. This provides her with adequate calcium to take care of her own needs as well as the needs of her unborn child.

Breast milk production requires about 160 to 300 milligrams of calcium per day, but overall, calcium needs during breastfeeding are similar to the needs during pregnancy. As such, the National Research Council has made the new recommendations for breastfeeding the same as those during pregnancy. Thus, a pregnant woman over the age of eighteen and a woman who is nursing should be getting 1,000 milligrams of calcium each day. The pregnant adolescent, however, has needs of her own and should continue to get 1,300 milligrams per day.

Calcium Recommendations for Infants and Young Children

Between the amount of calcium contained in breast milk and in formulas coupled with the enhanced calcium absorption that occurs during the first year of life, most healthy, full-term infants usually get an adequate supply of calcium. According to the DRIs, infants up to five months old should be receiving 210 milligrams and infants six to eleven months old should be receiving 270 milligrams of calcium per day.

Healthy infants absorb almost three-fourths of their calcium intake; however, premature babies or those who have special health problems need individualized recommendations from their healthcare professionals. The amount they need and their individual ability to use calcium will vary.

Calcium requirements for young children are based primarily on the needs for skeletal growth and bone mineralization. This is the time in life during which they are developing in bone length and strength to last a lifetime. A calcium deficiency during these crucial growing years could prevent them from reaching their potential adult height.

About two pounds of calcium are deposited in a child's skeleton between birth and adulthood. As children continue to grow and to form more bone, their calcium requirements also increase. Recommendations have been established by age group, which reflect their changing needs. Children one to three years old should be receiving 500 milligrams per day and children four to eight years old should be receiving 800 milligrams of calcium per day.

Calcium Recommendations for Adolescents and Young Adults

The daily accumulation of calcium in the skeleton around the time of puberty and during adolescence may be as high as 400 to 500 milligrams per day. Children begin to grow and change rapidly at this time. During adolescent years, boys on average grow six inches in height and gain about forty-five pounds. Girls grow about six inches and gain about thirty-five pounds.

Bone length and much of an adult's bone density—the amount of bone mineral content—will be attained largely by about twenty years of age, although additional bone mass continues to develop into the third decade of life. Studies have consistently shown that bone mass is increased by calcium intakes of around 1,200 milligrams per day, when accompanied by an adequate vitamin D intake.

Consequences of a deficient calcium intake during adolescence, particularly when children are inactive may seriously affect the amount of bone mineralization that occurs due to the rapid rate of growth that takes place. Accumulating maximum calcium stores in the skeleton during these young years is considered among the best protections against age-related bone loss and fractures in later life.

Although boys and girls grow to different heights and weights at widely varying rates, based on reviews of many studies, calcium intake recommendations have been divided by age, not sex. Adolescents nine to eighteen years old should be receiving 1,300 milligrams of calcium per day. Adolescents over eighteen years old and young adults should follow adult recommendations of 1,000 milligrams per day.

Calcium Recommendations for Peri- and Postmenopausal Women

As the average woman approaches the fifth decade of her life, her body undergoes numerous changes. Among the most notable is the dwindling production of the female hormones, estrogen and progesterone, which are known to be strong protectors of bone. This period of life is known as menopause, and the interim period during which this change is occurring is termed peri-menopause (meaning "around" the time of menopause). The peri-menopausal period may be brief or may take up to a few years, depending on the woman.

The diminished production of female hormones results in an almost inevitable rapid loss of bone, especially during the five years immediately following the cessation of menstruation—the traditional signal that hormone production is declining. Up until this time, female hormones have had powerful influences over bone health. Women who are fifty to sixty years of age may lose about 10 to 20 percent of their bone mass during these years. If a woman had maximized the accumulation of calcium in her bones during the years of bone formation, she will benefit by having more bone to lose. With more bone mass, she has a lower risk of suffering a fracture than the woman who had a lower or inadequate bone mass at the onset of menopause. In about ten years after the onset of menopause, bone loss stabilizes at about 1 percent per year.

However, at the time of menopause and beyond, sufficient calcium intake continues to be essential to help maintain calcium balance and help minimize additional bone loss. In contrast to the 1989 RDAs for which the calcium-intake recommendation was the same for everyone over fifty years old, the new DRIs provide calcium recommendations for men and women fifty-one to seventy years old and for those older than seventy. Unfortunately, the DRIs do not specifically address the needs of peri- and postmenopausal women.

In 1994, calcium experts at the National Institutes of Health Consensus Conference on Optimal Calcium Intake established two sets of recommendations for peri- and postmenopausal women. They recommended that women on hormone replacement therapy (HRT) get 1,000 milligrams of calcium per day. HRT, which is aimed at replacing a woman's own dwindling supply of female hormones, is a prescription medication that has been shown to very effectively limit the loss of bone in this group. But along with its bone benefits, as with any drug, HRT carries some health risks and is not appropriate for some women.

For women not on HRT, the committee recommended that postmenopausal women get 1,500 milligrams a day of calcium to help limit bone loss. But these calcium experts also cautioned that calcium intake alone should not be considered a replacement for HRT. A woman at this stage of life should consult with her health-care professional to discuss the best options for her.

Calcium Recommendations for Older Adults

As we age, the body's ability to handle calcium changes along with the amount of calcium that the body needs. These changes affect how much calcium may be absorbed and how much the body retains. Some of these changes are thought to begin as early as sixty years of age—particularly in postmenopausal women.

Generally, in later years, less stomach acid is produced, and in some cases, less calcium is absorbed. When the body senses that there's inadequate calcium, it signals the brain to secrete more parathyroid hormone (PTH). This causes calcium to be released from bone to maintain the level of calcium in the blood, as discussed in Chapter 2. Also, in later years, the body's ability to synthesize vitamin D becomes less efficient, which in turn creates an environment in the body whereby the kidneys more readily lose calcium. Taking all of these physical changes and other factors into consideration, it has been recommended that both men and women over fifty years old should increase their calcium intake to 1,200 milligrams each day.

Is There Such a Thing as Too Much Calcium?

Even a mineral as important as calcium has its upper limits of safety. For some vulnerable people, a calcium intake that is too high may lead to serious health problems and can even interfere with nutrition balance. Fortunately, most toxic effects associated with too much calcium seem to be rare. In 1997, based on a review of scientific studies, the Food and Nutrition Board set 2,500 milligrams of calcium per day as the *Tolerable Upper Intake Level*. This is the maximum amount of calcium that appears to be safe for most healthy Americans to consume on a regular basis.

We know that the need for calcium remains relatively high throughout life and that the body insures that, whenever it can, it gets its calcium by increasing the amount it absorbs. The body also has the ability to decrease the amount it absorbs, and excretes surplus calcium to lessen the chances of harm. This balancing act normally works very well, but it can be overridden. When calcium intake is about 4,000 milligrams per day or more, the body's ability to protect itself from retaining too much calcium may fail. Even at slightly lower intakes, certain people may experience adverse effects from too much calcium.

Most people consume far less than 4,000 milligrams of calcium per day or even the 2,500 milligrams upper limit that is advised: the median intake for adult women is slightly less than 600 milligrams per day and for men it is about 800 milligrams per day. But with increasing efforts to promote calcium-rich products like calcium-fortified beverages and breakfast cereals, and the escalating use of calcium supplements, there is probable cause for concern that there will be intentional as well as unintentional substantial increases in calcium that may be harmful.

Physiological Consequences of Excess Calcium

Much of what has been learned about the consequences of calcium toxicity is derived from various animal studies and human case reports. For example, Sarah is a fifty-year-old schoolteacher with three children. A thin woman, Sarah had a typical calcium intake for her group of about 700 milligrams per day and was concerned about her aging bones and the effect of menopause on her skeleton. So she switched to calcium-fortified orange juice at breakfast and lunch, she began eating calcium-fortified cereal at breakfast, and she started taking several calcium carbonate-containing antacids to get the rest of her calcium.

Out of the blue, Sarah began suffering weird, nonspecific, and debilitating symptoms like irritability, headaches, and constipation. Then suddenly she began to have sharp, strong pains similar to what she'd experienced when she had been suffering from kidney stones. A medical exam revealed that her blood calcium levels were elevated, she had too much calcium in her urine, her body's acidity level was out of balance, and she was having a recurrence of kidney stones. Sarah told her doctor that she'd been taking ten to twelve calcium-carbonate antacid tablets every day—amounting to more than 2,000 milligrams of calcium daily—in addition to having increased her calcium intake from foods. From an analysis of Sarah's diet, a dietitian determined that she was consuming more than 3,500 milligrams of calcium per day. See Table 8.2 on page 100 for an illustration of Sarah's diet and how easy it was for her calcium intake to accumulate.

Sarah was fortunate to have sought medical attention before too much time elapsed. When regular calcium intake is excessive, fatal kidney damage, sudden death, or a deposition of calcium into soft tissues, resulting in the hardening of some organs, may occur. After Sarah stopped taking the antacids and was given other medical treatment, her problems were resolved without permanent damage. She met again with her dietitian to learn how to properly balance her calcium intake with her individual needs. In her case, by eliminating the antacids alone, she found that she could meet her needs for calcium.

It's important to note that calcium toxicity is unlikely to occur from food intake alone. It was Sarah's naive use of supplemental calcium that had worked against her. Unless there are exceptional con-

TABLE 8.2. SARAH'S DIET BEFORE AND AFTER INCREASING HER CALCIUM INTAKE			
	Menu	Sarah's diet before increasing calcium intake	Sarah's diet after increasing calcium intake
Breakfast	Calcium-fortified Orange juice, 1 cup	22 mg (not fortified)	300 mg
	Calcium-fortified whole grain cereal, 1 cup	26 mg (not fortified)	200 mg
	Skim milk, 1 cup	300 mg	300 mg
Lunch	Cottage cheese, 1 cup	120 mg	120 mg
	Carrot sticks, ½ cup	9 mg	9 mg
	Whole wheat bread, 1 slice	25 mg	25 mg
	Peanut butter, 1 tbsp.	6 mg	6 mg
	Calcium-fortified orange juice	(not applicable)	300 mg
	Banana	7 mg	7 mg
Dinner	Salmon fillet, 4 oz.	17 mg	17 mg
	Buttered brown rice, 1 cup	20 mg	20 mg
	Broccoli, 1 cup	75 mg	75 mg
	Garlic French bread, 1 slice	26 mg	26 mg
	Water	0 mg	0 mg
	Brownie	11 mg	11 mg
	Calcium-carbonate antacids (each 250 mg calcium)	(not applicable)	2,500 mg
Total calcium		664 mg	3,916 mg

ditions, science, as well as common sense, dictates that wholesome, unrefined food should be the first choice for optimizing calcium intake.

Nutritional Consequences of Excess Calcium

Naively increasing calcium intake to excess levels can upset the body's nutritional balance, which is necessary for optimal functioning. For example, overindulging in traditional dairy foods to increase calcium intake can result in an increase in the amount of saturated fat that is consumed, unless low-fat or nonfat dairy foods are used. Focusing primarily on calcium-fortified juices for calcium and limiting the intake of calcium-rich vegetables will likely result in a low intake of dietary fiber and phytochemicals.

In addition, a surplus intake of calcium may override the body's ability to absorb optimum amounts of some minerals, such as iron, magnesium, and zinc, which could contribute to a potential deficiency. This is because the presence of calcium can upset the balance in the intestinal tract necessary for the absorption of some other minerals. In those who already have a poor intake of some nutrients, such as children and the elderly, this situation is of special concern.

Some Final Words

Clearly, moderation and balance are chief factors for optimizing calcium's usefulness to the body. As with most nutrients in the body, there is a point where calcium's powerful influences can be harmful rather than being beneficial. At present, extensive, long-term knowledge about the potential harmful effects of excess calcium is relatively unknown, since a calcium deficiency is so much more common. Research will continue to fill in the pieces of information that are missing. In the meantime, it comes down to that old maxim—*moderation in all things.*

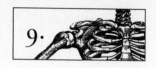

Food Sources of Calcium

To SATISFY the body's requirements and to protect the bones and teeth, calcium is needed in relatively large amounts each day. The newly released Dietary Reference Intakes discussed in the previous chapter provide us with the latest recommendations about how much calcium we should be consuming. The next step is to find out how to go about getting the right amounts of calcium from the foods that we eat.

In the American tradition, milk is almost universally considered to be an indispensable calcium source. Without it, we are led to believe that our intake of calcium would fall short. However, not all experts agree with this conventional opinion. So, when it comes to choosing calcium-rich foods, extend your thinking beyond that traditional glass of milk. Rich sources of calcium are found in many other dairy foods, like yogurt, kefir, and cheese. Less familiar, but well worth the effort, is to obtain some of your daily calcium from plant foods, such as calcium-fortified plant-based beverages, some kinds of nuts, and vegetables.

Dairy Foods and Calcium Intake—
A Modern Tradition

Milk drinking by contemporary humans is a very modern tradition. Although dairy products enjoy extensive popularity almost world-wide, drinking milk past infancy is the exception rather than the rule in the mammalian kingdom. Even in the earliest history of human beings, only infants consumed milk and that was during breast-feeding. Our hunter-gatherer ancestors got their calcium from naturally occurring, wholesome foods that came directly from nature. Studies of the fossilized remains of food and other artifacts of early humans have revealed that for many thousands of years, they consumed a calcium-rich diet, comprised primarily of wild game—which possibly included consuming some of the calcium-rich bones of their kill—and uncultivated, wild plants.

The custom of milk drinking by humans other than infants began with animal husbandry, but only after we had developed the ability to keep milk from spoiling. Before refrigeration, milk spoiled rapidly in warm climates. Humans discovered almost certainly by accident that the resulting curdled or fermented product remained edible for a much longer period of time than did fresh milk. Humans have since relied on the fermentation process to preserve milk, which gives us yogurt, kefir, koumiss (made from camel's, mare's, or cow's milk), and cheese. Compare the expiration date on a container of yogurt with the date on a carton of milk purchased at the same time. You'll see that the yogurt will remain edible much longer.

Thus, the modern tradition of relying on milk drinking as our primary source of dietary calcium is not based on biological history, but is instead linked, in part, to its improved availability due to modern technology.

Modern Day Dairy Sources of Calcium

Dairy foods—with exception of those products consisting chiefly of dairy fat, like butter, cream, sour cream, and cream cheese—continue to be the top choices of dietary calcium for Americans. Although milk typically is thought of as the richest source of calcium, some fermented dairy products, like yogurt, can actually supply more calcium for the same amount of calories. A cup of plain nonfat yogurt provides as much as 450 milligrams of calcium and about 90 calories, while 8 ounces of nonfat milk contains, on average, 290 milligrams of calcium and about the same amount of calories as the yogurt.

Calcium-rich dairy foods are also high in protein and phosphorus in naturally balanced amounts and are also good sources of other nutrients, including riboflavin, niacin, vitamin B_{12}, and magnesium.

Adults get close to 70 percent of their calcium from dairy products, whereas children get up to 75 percent. Together, milk and cheese account for 60 percent of our total daily dietary calcium, with the average person eating about 27 pounds of cheese a year or just over 1 ounce per day. See Figure 9.1 on page 105, which illustrates the major sources of calcium in the American diet.

Throughout the world, calcium from dairy foods is obtained from a wide variety of animal species. In the United States, most dairy foods come from cows, followed by goats. In other countries, fermented milk products such as yogurt and milk from buffaloes, sheep, and goats supply most of the calcium. Dairy foods from donkeys, horses, oxen, and reindeer are also consumed but to a much lesser extent.

Top Dairy Choices for Calcium

Fermented or cultured dairy foods like yogurt are excellent calcium-rich choices for almost everyone. These products have been part of

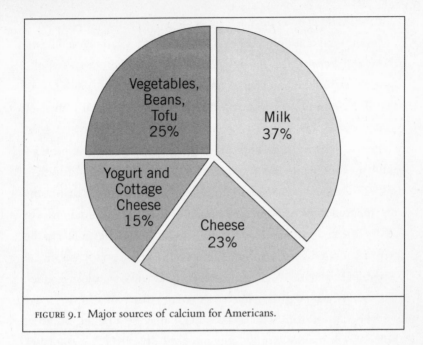

FIGURE 9.1 Major sources of calcium for Americans.

the human diet longer than fresh milk has and for about as long as cheese. Among the other top sources of calcium-rich dairy foods are cow's milk and goat's milk, which are the two most commonly consumed varieties of fresh milk in the United States. Cheese is also popular throughout many parts of the world, and there are over a thousand calcium-rich cheeses from which to choose.

Yogurt Yogurt can be made from any kind of mammalian milk. In some parts of the world, the native yogurt of the region has been esteemed for its health benefits for centuries. However, it was not until the second half of the twentieth century that yogurt caught on in the United States. Since then, the rise in yogurt's popularity has been phenomenal. In addition to its high calcium content, yogurt is a very appealing, nutritious food that is easier than fresh milk for some people to digest. Its nutritional value is nearly the same as that of the kind of mammalian milk from which it is made.

Yogurt probably originated from leaving milk out in warm temperatures, where inherent bacteria acted on the milk. Today, carefully controlled conditions are used. Bacteria, usually *Lactobacillis bulgaricus* and *Streptococcus thermophilus,* are added to either whole, low-fat, or nonfat milk. The bacteria transform some of the sugar in the milk, lactose, into a waste product called lactic acid. It is the lactic acid that gives yogurt its characteristic tangy flavor and contributes to its easy digestibility. In addition, the kind of proteins found in yogurt are also thought to be more easily digested than milk, since they tend to break down faster in the stomach than some unfermented milk proteins. Although the calcium content is not usually affected, yogurt made with low-fat or whole milk can be high in saturated fat. Also, depending on the brand and flavor, it can be high in sweeteners and other added ingredients, thus losing much of its traditional yogurt character. A yogurt that contains the active bacteria cultures from which it was made may be a better, healthier choice. Look for the words "contains active bacteria" on the label, along with a minimal amount of added sweeteners or other added ingredients.

Yogurt Cheese Yogurt can be made into a soft and creamy textured food that resembles cream cheese and has a slightly tangy flavor. It is a particularly concentrated source of calcium that supplies nearly 500 milligrams of calcium per cup, with the same digestive benefits as regular yogurt.

Any kind of plain yogurt that does not contain gelatin or gums can be used. Many people prefer the richer flavor and consistency of yogurt cheese that has been made from low-fat or whole milk, rather than nonfat milk. However, there will be some extra calories and fat—just as you would get from using low-fat or whole milk instead of nonfat milk. Unfortunately, yogurt cheese is not usually available on the market shelf, but it is simple to prepare, since it essentially makes itself. See the inset "Recipe for Yogurt Cheese" on page 107.

Recipe for Yogurt Cheese

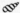

Yogurt cheese is a rich source of calcium that practically makes itself overnight. Each cup will supply nearly 500 milligrams of calcium. Use it as spread on toast, to mix with your favorite seasonings for a vegetable dip, or top it with honey and nuts for a quick lunch or snack.

Take one quart (4 cups) of plain nonfat or low-fat yogurt without added gelatin or gums. Line a strainer large enough to hold the yogurt with a double thickness of wet cheesecloth. Place the strainer in a bowl that is shaped to prevent the yogurt from sitting in the liquid that will drain from it. Spoon the yogurt into the strainer, fold the end of the cheesecloth over the top of the yogurt, and allow the liquid to drain into the bowl. Be sure that the bottom of the strainer does not touch the liquid. Refrigerate overnight.

The next day, check the yogurt for desired thickness—leave longer until it is as thick as you desire. Then, scoop the cheese out of the strainer and store it in a sealed container. Discard the liquid. Yogurt cheese keeps for about two weeks refrigerated.

Kefir Kefir is a yogurt-like beverage, also sometimes known as "liquid yogurt." In Southwestern Asia, it originally was made from camel's milk. It also can be made from the milk of cows, goats, or mares. Today, kefir from cow's milk is most common.

Kefir is made by a double fermentation process using bacteria and yeast. Kefir is slightly fizzy and has been described as having a slightly piquant, sour flavor and has a 1 to 2 percent alcohol content due to fermentation. Being similar to yogurt, the lactose has been partially digested, so people who cannot tolerate lactose can often enjoy kefir with less or no discomfort. It usually is found in specialty shops and health food stores. One cup provides about 300 milligrams of calcium.

Cow's Milk As a traditional calcium-rich source, cow's milk finds its way into most homes. For adults and children over two years old, nonfat milk is the best choice with 1 percent low-fat being the next best. This is because low-fat (both 1 percent and 2 percent low-fat milks) and whole milk are high in saturated fat. Note, however, that children younger than age two need the calories that whole milk or formulas provide, as advised by a pediatrician, to support their growth and development. They should not be given low-fat or nonfat milk.

Milk in the United States is fortified with vitamin D. As you learned in Chapter 6, vitamin D helps the body to absorb calcium. Note that most other dairy foods do not have added vitamin D, unless they were prepared with vitamin D-fortified milk.

Goat's Milk Goat's milk has been an important source of calcium for humans for hundreds of years. Goat's milk provides more calcium and less cholesterol than its bovine counterpart. Its fat and protein makeup also is somewhat different and may be easier to digest than cow's milk. People who are allergic to cow's milk can sometimes tolerate goat's milk without ill effects because of the differences in the protein makeup.

Goat's milk baby formulas are among the practical alternatives for infants who are unable to tolerate cow's milk formulas. In fact, physicians have recommended goat's milk formula for infant patients since the time of Hippocrates. Milk from goats, though, like cow's milk, contains lactose, so someone who is lactose intolerant may experience similar digestive difficulties. (See Lactose Intolerance on page 111.)

Cheese The world of cheese is a delightful place that has long been romanticized, and humans have had a long and great love affair with it. Cheese made from goat's milk has been common since ancient Roman times and was known as the foods of gods and heroes in mythology. There are over a thousand varieties of cheese worldwide.

Since it takes about 11 pounds of milk to make 1 pound of cheese, many cheeses are loaded with calcium. But bear in mind that cheese and calcium do not always go hand in hand. The calcium-richness of a cheese will vary depending on a number of factors, including the type of milk used and the method of production.

Among the cheeses with the most calcium are Romano and Parmesan, containing about 300 milligrams per ounce. One ounce (about the size of a one-inch cube) of popular aged-cheeses like Cheddar or Monterey Jack will supply about 200 milligrams of calcium. But cottage cheese is much lower in calcium when compared with them. It takes about two cups of low-fat cottage cheese to come close to the calcium in one ounce of aged Cheddar or Monterey Jack.

For the calcium it provides, cheese made from whole milk is also very high in saturated fat. When it comes to the popular cheeses, like Cheddar, Monterey Jack, or Swiss, lower fat or fat-free varieties are worth exploring. Alternatively, try turning to soy cheeses that have been fortified with calcium. Although they may have similar amounts of fat, the fat is unsaturated, which is a good, heart-healthy type of fat.

Not All Dairy Is Calcium-Rich

Some dairy foods have essentially zero calcium: cream cheese, sour cream, cream, and butter are among them. You would need to eat more than one cup of cream cheese to get the same amount of calcium in one cup of yogurt at almost ten times the calories. A cup of nonfat yogurt has about 90 calories, but a cup of cream cheese contains more than 800 calories—not to mention close to 100 grams of fat. Frozen treats like ice cream also supply very little calcium comparably speaking—especially when calories and fat are taken into account.

When Dairy Products Don't Agree with Your Body

Not everyone is born with or, past infancy, is able to tolerate some dairy products. A small proportion of adults and children have a true milk allergy, and the majority of the world population's ability to digest lactose, a sugar in milk, declines to about 5 to 10 percent from infancy.

Milk Allergies

A true milk allergy involves activation of the body's immune system. It occurs when a protein found in milk, like casein, lactalglobulin, or lactalbumin, is absorbed intact without first being digested into the bloodstream. This causes the release of antibodies and other defensive agents into the bloodstream. Milk is believed to be one of the most common of all food allergies and tends to run in families. Cow's milk is generally a frequent offender due to its high level of consumption especially in infants and children, although other kinds of milk may also elicit an allergic reaction. Although allergies can appear at any age, they are most common during the first few years of life. As children grow, typically they become less sensitive to the offending food. However, the tendency may never become completely outgrown.

A true milk allergy results in a large variety of symptoms that can occur within minutes or several hours after drinking milk or eating a food that contains milk proteins. Allergic symptoms can range from hives, sneezing, runny or stuffy nose, and intestinal problems that include nausea, vomiting, and diarrhea. In extreme cases, severe reactions such as swelling of the throat or tongue, and breathing problems such as asthma may occur. Without proper medical treatment, a person experiencing such a reaction is in danger of dying. People who are very sensitive to cow's milk proteins need to turn to sources other than dairy for their calcium.

Lactose Intolerance

Lactose intolerance develops when the body loses its ability to break down some or all of the lactose, a sugar found in milk. Since early in the twentieth century, it has been known that lactose appears to help the body absorb calcium, especially in infants. However, lactose intolerance prevents many people from being able to enjoy milk and some other dairy foods. Lactose is unique in the world of sugars, because it is the only animal-derived sugar—all other sugars in nature come from plants. The only non-animal sources of lactose are found in trace amounts in forsythia flowers and a few tropical plants.

Lactose is a dissacharide, a sugar molecule comprised of two single sugars—in this case, they are glucose and galactose. Lactose must be broken down in the digestive tract into its single sugar units before it can be absorbed and used by the body. Digestion of lactose requires the activity of the enzyme lactase. When the body produces no or insufficient amounts of lactase, a person is lactose intolerant.

Lactose intolerance was once thought to be a medical deficiency, but it is now known that family history plays a large part. Lactose intolerance also may develop as a consequence of certain medical conditions such as intestinal disease or stomach surgery, or from use of some medications such as the antibiotics neomycin and kanamycin—which reduce lactase production. Losing most or all of the ability to digest lactose is considered to be a normal physiological change for much of the world's population after infancy. In fact, this loss is normal in all other mammals.

Most people produce the most lactase during infancy, when they are relying on breast milk or formula. But by early adulthood, the ability to digest lactose may drop by as much as 95 percent. Because family history plays a big role, this doesn't happen to everyone. However, throughout the world, only about 30 percent of the population retains the ability to digest large amounts of lactose.

When more lactose is consumed than can be handled by the body, it is left undigested and passes directly to the colon. Bacteria in the colon then ferment the lactose, which produces uncomfortable symptoms like intestinal gas, bloating, abdominal distention, and diarrhea. The number and severity of symptoms that occur can vary widely among individuals. Some people can handle some lactose—that is, they produce some lactase—and tend to experience fewer problems if they consume small amounts of lactose-containing foods throughout the day or consume the lactose-containing foods as part of a mixed meal. Others cannot handle even small amounts of lactose, because they produce no lactase whatsoever and, therefore, must find other sources of calcium.

Unfermented dairy foods, like milk—whether whole, low-fat or nonfat—contain large amounts of lactose. Prepared foods containing milk solids, even those that are labeled non-dairy, may contain lactose. Baked and processed foods like breads, cereals, cold cuts, salad dressings, sauces, gravies, or candies may contain lactose. When the terms dry milk solids, malted milk, sour or sweet cream, whey, cheese, or lactose appear on the ingredient list on a food label, the product contains lactose. Someone who is extremely lactose intolerant needs to check food labels carefully. Even some medications may contain lactose. Consult with your health-care professional about appropriate medications.

Most fermented or cultured calcium-rich dairy products, like yogurt, kefir, and buttermilk made with active cultures (check the label—not all cultured dairy foods contains live cultures) and acidophilus milks are good alternatives because some or all of the lactose has already been broken down to glucose and galactose. Aged cheeses, like Cheddar, Monterey Jack, Swiss, and Parmesan also contain less lactose than fresh milk because the liquid whey portion of milk—which contains the lactose—is removed during the cheese-making process. The longer that a cheese is aged, the less lactose it usually contains.

As another option, special products have been developed for people with lactose intolerance. Some products have had the lactose reduced. Others, like tablets that are taken before consuming lactose-containing foods, contain lactase. In addition, there are calcium-fortified, non-dairy beverages, including rice milks, soymilks, and nut milks, which contain no lactose at all. If you are lactose intolerant, be sure that you are getting enough calcium from alternative sources.

Non-Dairy Animal-Based Calcium Sources

Most non-dairy animal foods such as meats, fish, and poultry contain so little calcium that they're not worth mentioning as calcium sources. However, there are two exceptions: canned sardines and canned salmon, which both contain edible bones that crumble easily. Three ounces of canned sardines supply about 324 milligrams of calcium, which is about the same or slightly more than you would get from an 8-ounce glass of milk. And three ounces of canned salmon yields about 312 milligrams of calcium.

Another animal-based source of calcium comes from a traditional method of preparing soup by Southeast Asians. They make a high-calcium stock by soaking cracked animal bones in vinegar and then boiling them in the vinegar until the bones turn soft and spongy. Due to the vinegar's acidity, the bones release their calcium into the liquid. One tablespoon of this stock may contain as much as

100 milligrams of calcium. In ancient times, other people, like those from the Mediterranean regions, soaked eggshells in lemon juice or vinegar to release the rich source of calcium in the shell.

Beyond Tradition—Getting Calcium from Plants

There are numerous foods outside of the animal kingdom that are high in calcium—although until now they have been largely unappreciated. When diets are based on plant foods, not only do they provide highly absorbable sources of calcium, but also a wealth of other protective substances. Also, relatively new calcium-fortified products, such as beverages, breads, and cereals are now available to help us meet our calcium needs.

The kingdom of plants offers a bountiful array of choices to help round out our calcium intake. Some plants supply significant amounts of calcium without the calcium-robbing proteins found in animal foods. In addition to calcium, numerous plant-food compounds called phytochemicals have been linked with a lower risk of degenerative diseases, such as cancer and heart disease. So it seems that our parents were right when they told us to eat our vegetables!

Non-Dairy Calcium-Fortified Beverages

In recent years, the popularity of plant-based beverages has escalated because of their taste and nutritional appeal. These beverages, including rice milk, soymilk, and nut milk, contain none of the saturated fat or cholesterol that is inherent in low-fat or whole milk calcium-rich dairy products. Unfortunately, these milks are not naturally high in calcium content, so they are often fortified with calcium and other nutrients. When choosing one of these beverages, check the label to insure that it lists calcium as one of the ingredients.

Also, it is important to emphasize that these kinds of beverages are inappropriate infant formula or breast milk alternatives for infants or children under two years of age. To grow and develop properly, they require large amounts of fat, as well as the calories and nutrients that are in specially prepared formulas or breast milk. Be sure to seek your pediatrician's guidance.

Rice Milk As a non-dairy beverage, calcium-fortified rice milk is a good option for those who do not wish to drink animal-based milks or those who would simply like some variety. It also is a suitable alternative for those who are allergic to cow's milk or soymilk or those who are lactose intolerant (see page 111). Usually made from brown rice and available plain or flavored, rice milk is fortified with calcium and vitamins A and D in amounts similar to that provided by cow's milk. (Be sure to read the ingredient listing on the label to insure that the product contains these nutrients.)

Almond Milk Made from real almonds and available in plain or flavored forms, almond milk is a great way to increase your variety of calcium-rich food choices. Almond milk is lactose-free and is fortified with vitamins A and D and additional calcium. Almonds naturally contain some calcium—see page 59—but additional calcium is added to make the level comparable to other similar products. If you can't find almond milk in your local market, ask your grocer to order it for you. Or if you are feeling enterprising, it is simple to make—although it won't be as high in calcium and won't contain vitamins A or D. See the inset "Making Nut Milks" on page 116.

Soymilk Most Asians have been enjoying soymilk for centuries. Made from crushed, cooked soybeans, soymilk is available plain or flavored and in low-fat and nonfat versions. However, some flavored soymilks can be high in calories from added sweeteners. Similar to rice and nut milks, soymilk contains no lactose, and the protein in

---

Making Nut Milks

☙

Even though their use goes back to ancient times, plant-based milks are only now increasing in popularity as highly nutritious contemporary options to traditional animal-based milk. Not only are some nut milks good sources of calcium—namely those made from almonds and hazelnuts—but they also supply us with numerous disease-fighting phytochemicals.

To make about one cup of nut milk, you need one cup of whole natural or blanched nuts—do not use roasted or salted nuts—and about three to four ice cubes. Place nuts in a food processor with a metal blade. Place ice cubes in a measuring cup and add enough water to make 1¼ cups. Pour the ice water into the food processor with the nuts. Add sweetenings, such as honey, if desired. Process until nuts and ice cubes are finely crushed. Strain the mixture through a double-thickness of cheesecloth, allowing the liquid to accumulate in a bowl. Squeeze out the remaining moisture from the mixture. Transfer the milk to a suitable container. Store in refrigerator for up to one week.

If you have a high power blender, it's even easier to make nut milk since no straining is required. Place the same amount of nuts, water, and ice cubes in the jar and cover. Blend first on low power then on high power until the mixture is liquefied. Add sweetening such as honey if desired.

---

soy has been found to help lower blood cholesterol levels. Soy also contains important phytochemicals called phytoestrogens. Early research suggests that these compounds may be protective against heart disease, bone loss, and some cancers.

Some individuals may be sensitive or allergic to soy, although true food allergies in general tend to be relatively rare, affecting fewer than 2 percent of adults and about 6 percent of children. Children are much more likely to experience allergies, and an allergy to soy is often outgrown. A true soy allergy will cause the same kinds of changes in the body's immune system as a true milk allergy (see page 110). If you experience allergic reactions such as runny nose, itchy skin, a rapid heartbeat, problems breathing, intestinal gas, vomiting, or diarrhea, seek advice from your health-care professional as soon as possible. Note that soy is found under several different guises and not always in recognizable terms. In addition to soymilk, soy concentrate, protein, and flour, soy is contained in hydrolyzed vegetable protein, textured vegetable protein (TVP), and vegetable protein concentrate—ingredients that are commonly added to convenient and processed foods.

The Calcium Power of Plants

For too many people, plant foods are highly unappreciated sources of calcium. Many varieties provide us with highly absorbable calcium, as well as with many other healthful and protective phytochemicals. In addition, plant foods contain no cholesterol or, with few exceptions, any saturated fats. Moreover, the proteins in plants contribute little to the potential calcium-draining effect for which animal proteins are known. And, for the most part, plants are lower in calories than their animal counterparts.

Leafy Greens Many members of the cabbage family are excellent, highly absorbable sources of calcium. Broccoli, Brussels sprouts, green cabbage, kale, turnip, collard greens, mustard greens, and kohlrabi—a member of the turnip family, also known as a cabbage turnip—are included in this calcium harvest. We also know that some varieties of seaweed, like nori—the popular seaweed used in making sushi rolls—are rich in calcium. Bok choy, the popular Chinese cabbage, is especially high in calcium. The body absorbs calcium from these foods just as well as, if not better than, it does from dairy foods. See the inset "Calcium Absorption of Selected Foods" below.

But not all leafy greens contain calcium that is highly absorbable. Traditionally, spinach, Swiss chard, and rhubarb have been widely promoted as good sources of calcium. While it is true that they con-

---

Calcium Absorption of Selected Foods

Some plant foods are better sources of useable calcium than milk, the most popular and widely consumed calcium source. The listing below ranks selected foods according to the amount of absorbable calcium they provide.

50 Percent or More Useable Calcium

- Bok choy
- Broccoli
- Brussels sprouts
- Cabbage
- Cauliflower
- Kale
- Kohlrabi
- Mustard greens
- Radish
- Rutabaga
- Turnip greens
- Watercress

20 to 35 Percent Absorbable Calcium

- Yogurt
- Milk
- Fortified soymilk, orange juice, and tofu

15 to 20 Percent Absorbable Calcium

- Almonds
- Beans

5 Percent or Less Absorbable Calcium

- Spinach
- Rhubarb
- Swiss Chard

tain ample amounts of calcium, the calcium they contain is poorly absorbed. This is because of the calcium-blocking action of the ox-alic acids contained in these greens. (Oxalic acid was discussed in Chapter 7.) But don't be too concerned. You would have to eat enormous amounts of these foods at the exclusion of all other calcium-rich foods for consumption of these greens to affect cal-cium nutrition.

Also, these leafy greens are extremely nutritious in their own right. They contain abundant amounts of other vitamins, minerals, and phytochemicals—all of which are important to good health and disease prevention. Despite their lack of absorbable calcium, they deserve some plate space in everyone's diet.

Fruit In contrast to some vegetables, most fruits contain little calcium. But outside of the daily garden variety of fruits, there are a few unique and interesting options that can contribute nicely to our overall calcium intake and dietary variety. One such fruit is the dried fig. Three dried figs will provide about 100 milligrams of calcium—which is about a tenth of an adult's daily recommendation. You may associate figs with cookies. But unfortunately, the amount of cal-cium in one of those cookies is so little that it is hardly worth men-tioning.

On the more exotic side, a tropical cherimoya, also known as a custard apple, yields about 125 milligrams of calcium, while the sapote will give you about 90 milligrams. Both the cherimoya and sapote are known for their creamy, custard-like textures when ripe. The cherimoya has the delicate flavors of pineapple, papaya, and ba-nana, and the sapote is sweetly suggestive of a peach-avocado-vanilla blend. Both can be found in specialty grocery stores and produce markets.

Nuts Too often ignored and too long vilified because of their high-fat content, research is confirming what ancient civilizations had known well. Nuts are among the best healthful kinds of foods that nature provides. They are high in minerals and vitamins, such as vitamin E, which may act to protect the body's cells from damage. They are rich in magnesium, one of calcium's close partners. Nuts are also abundant in many phytochemicals, which have been shown to be protective against some degenerative diseases, like heart disease and cancer. Nuts are high in arginine, an amino acid (a building block of protein) that recent research suggests may be important in helping to prevent heart disease. And the dietary fibers contained in nuts help keep bowel movements regular and may contribute to lowering cholesterol. Finally, the highly criticized fat in nuts is unsaturated, and several studies have indicated that they are beneficial in reducing the risk of heart disease by lowering blood cholesterol levels.

In terms of their calcium content, two kinds of nuts stand out. An ounce of almonds or hazelnuts (about ¼ cup of each) supplies nearly 100 milligrams of calcium for roughly 200 calories. Other nuts contain only small amounts of calcium. Sprinkling some almonds or hazelnuts on a salad or a bowl of pasta and replacing chips or crackers with a small handful of nuts as a snack are quick and easy ways to add some nutty sources of calcium to your diet. Almond milk (see page 115) is another option for increasing nut intake. However, you will lose some of the nutritious goodness, like the fat and fiber, if you do not eat the pulp along with the milk.

Legumes Many kinds of cooked dry beans—like pinto, black, kidney, or garbanzo beans—contain some calcium. They also contain beneficial plant proteins, vitamins, minerals, dietary fiber, and phytochemicals. As with nuts, beans can be added to salads and pasta dishes. Or try adding some to soups and stews.

A legume-based food that is deserving of special attention is that 2,000-year-old ancient food, tofu, also known as soybean curd. Tofu is made from soymilk that has been extracted from ground, cooked soybeans and coagulated or set with a salt, such as calcium chloride, calcium sulfate, or magnesium sulfate. Sometimes an acid, like vinegar or lemon juice, may be used. Calcium-set tofu is an easily digestible and well-absorbed source of calcium at a relatively low calorie cost. Tofu absorbs the flavors with which it is prepared and lends itself to a wide variety of preparation methods. Try adding some small tofu cubes to soups or scrambled eggs, or add some tofu to your next meat-based stir-fry.

In addition to being an excellent source of protein and unsaturated, heart-healthy fats, one cup of tofu made with calcium (check the ingredient listing to be sure it is made with calcium) will provide you with about 260 milligrams of calcium for only 180 calories.

Calcium and Food Processing

As nutrition experts and the general public are increasingly recognizing calcium's health benefits, food manufacturers have begun to intentionally add calcium to foods to increase their calcium content. Calcium-fortified beverages, like juices, waters, and sports drinks, and breakfast cereals are now widely available and are rich sources of calcium. But some of these beverages and cereals may also be high in sugar due to added sweeteners. Calcium also finds it way into foods unintentionally during some food-processing practices. It gets into canned tomatoes due to firming agents that are added and into stone-ground flour from the limestone rock used in the grinding process. Also, as sugar is concentrated to form the very thick and dark colored blackstrap molasses, calcium content increases.

Getting the Most Calcium Power from Food

Insuring that we consume ample calcium means not only choosing foods that are high in calcium, but also finding calcium-rich foods that will meet our personal preferences and fit permanently into our unique lifestyles. The most benefit will be gained by consuming calcium-rich foods that we enjoy and are motivated to eat. This will lessen the chances of returning to a diet low in calcium. There is a wealth of calcium-rich foods from which to choose. The greater the variety we have, the more likely we are to benefit.

Focusing on variety helps to maintain interest and increases the ability to maintain a high calcium diet. It is very easy to become bored when you eat the same foods day in and day out—especially when you do so because it's "for your own good" and not because of preference. Eventually, you will get frustrated and slowly return to your old eating habits. To help insure your success, experiment with some of the calcium-rich foods that are new to you. When you think calcium, think variety.

Choosing Foods with the Most Calcium Power

When choosing calcium-rich foods, it's important to make the kinds of choices that will maximize calcium intake within a balance of other things, like calories and saturated fat. A key to this dilemma is finding those foods that have the most calcium for the amount of calories they provide.

To choose foods with the most calcium power, start by reviewing Table 9.1 on page 123. Calcium power is the amount of calcium relative to calorie content. To figure out the calcium power of a food not shown in the table, you need to know two things: the amount of calcium the food contains and the calories per serving. If you don't have a food label to follow, this information can be found in books on food composition or on nutrition-related computer software programs.

Food labels provide the calcium content of a food as a percentage of the U.S. Food and Drug Administration (FDA) recommended daily values (DV). The DV for calcium is 1,000 milligrams. To get the calcium content in milligrams of a food that contains 30 percent of the DV for calcium, you need to convert the percentage to decimals (30 percent would be .30) and then multiply it by 100. (.30 multiplied by 100 equals 300, or 300 milligrams of calcium.)

Now, to get the calcium power of a food, divide the amount of calcium it contains by its calories. For example, one cup of nonfat yogurt has 120 calories and the calcium content is 40 percent of the DV, or 400 milligrams. Divide the calcium content by the number of calories it contains. (400 divided by 120 equals a calcium power of

TABLE 9.1. CALCIUM POWER OF SELECTED FOODS			
Food	Calories	Calcium	Calcium Power
Beverages			
Buttermilk, nonfat or skim, 1 cup	100	280 mg	2.8
Cow's milk, 2 percent or low-fat, 1 cup	120	300 mg	2.5
Cow's milk, chocolate, 1 percent fat	160	290 mg	1.8
Cow's milk, nonfat or skim, 1 cup	90	300 mg	3.3
Cow's milk, whole, 1 cup	150	290 mg	1.9
Goat's milk, 1 cup	170	325 mg	1.9
Rice milk, calcium-fortified, plain, 1 cup	120	300 mg	2.5
Sheep milk, 1 cup	265	470 mg	1.8
Soymilk, nonfat, calcium-fortified, 1 cup	80	200 mg	2.5
Fermented Dairy Foods			
Kefir, 2 percent or low-fat, 1 cup	120	350 mg	2.9
Yogurt, plain, low-fat, 1 cup	144	415 mg	2.9
Yogurt, plain, nonfat, 1 cup	120	350 mg	2.9
Yogurt, plain, whole milk, 1 cup	296	150 mg	0.51
Selected Cheeses			
American cheese spread, 1 ounce	80	170 mg	2.13
Cottage cheese, 2 percent or low-fat, 1 cup	200	155 mg	0.78
Cottage cheese, nonfat, 1 cup	160	120 mg	0.75
Goat cheese, hard, 1 ounce	130	250 mg	1.9
Goat cheese, soft type, 1 ounce	75	40 mg	0.53

Hard cheese (Cheddar, Monterey Jack) 1 ounce	120	200 mg	1.7
Mozzarella, part-skim, 1 ounce	80	200 mg	2.5
Parmesan cheese, grated, 1 tablespoon	120	390 mg	3.3
Romano cheese, grated, 1 tablespoon	120	390 mg	3.3
Swiss, 1 ounce	110	270 mg	2.5
Yogurt cheese, nonfat, 1 cup	170	450 mg	2.7

Other Dairy Foods

Butter, 1 teaspoon	35	1 mg	0.03
Cream cheese, 2 tablespoons	99	23 mg	0.23
Half and half, 2 tablespoons	40	32 mg	0.80
Ice cream, ½ cup	170	87 mg	0.51
Sour cream, 2 tablespoons	52	28 mg	0.54

Other Animal-Based Foods

Beef, lamb, pork, veal, poultry, cooked, 3 ounces	200	16 mg	0.08
Hot dogs (Beef and Pork)	180	6 mg	0.03
Luncheon meat, 1 slice	51	2 mg	0.04
Salmon, canned with bones, 3 ounces	120	212 mg	1.8
Sardines, canned with bones, 3 ounces	177	324 mg	1.8

Vegetables

Almonds, ¼ cup	200	94 mg	0.47
Beet greens, cooked, 1 cup	40	164 mg	4.1
Bok choy, cooked, 1 cup	20	160 mg	8.0
Broccoli, cooked, 1 cup	56	178 mg	3.2
Brussels sprouts, cooked, 1 cup	61	56 mg	0.92
Cabbage, green or red, cooked, 1 cup	33	50 mg	1.5
Collard greens, cooked, 1 cup	54	298 mg	5.5
Kale, cooked, 1 cup	42	94 mg	2.2
Kohlrabi, cooked, 1 cup	48	41 mg	0.85
Mustard greens, cooked, 1 cup	22	104 mg	4.7
Nori, 3.5 ounces	35	70 mg	2.0
Pinto beans, cooked, 1 cup	234	82 mg	0.35
Tofu, calcium-set, ½ cup	183	258 mg	1.4

3.3.) This means that for every calorie, you're getting approximately 3 milligrams of calcium.

As you can see from Table 9.1, the best animal-based calcium source is yogurt with the highest calcium power of 2.9. Yogurt is available in many different ways to please almost anyone's palate. It's delicious with the addition of fruit or can be combined with cucumbers, garlic, and salt—a traditional Greek dish called tzatziki. Also, there are many brands of yogurt that are already flavored and ready for eating. Nonfat milk, which is low in calories and fat, and some cheeses are among the richest animal-based sources of calcium power.

As you read down the column of calcium-rich vegetables, it is apparent that bok choy, collard greens, and mustard greens are extraordinarily high in calcium. Broccoli, kale, nori, and cabbage aren't far behind. Nearly all these vegetables lend themselves to a wide range of opportunities to be included in your daily meals. All of the greens, including kale and broccoli are especially colorful additions to pasta and risotto dishes as well as to soups and stews. Particularly when cut into thin shreds, the greens lend an enticing green striping to these types of dishes and are especially appetizing when red pepper or tomatoes are used to add more color. In addition, there are literally hundreds of recipes that include more than one of these calcium-rich sources—especially look for traditional Asian, Middle Eastern, or Mediterranean-style recipes to add something new to your high calcium-way of eating.

Fifty Ways to Get More Calcium

Knowing that we need calcium every day and how much is found in typical foods is a good way to begin. But getting started is often another matter. Here are fifty ideas for adding calcium power to your daily meals:

1. Increase the calcium power of milk by adding powdered milk to your fresh milk. A quarter cup of powdered milk added to a quart of milk provides over 350 milligrams additional calcium per quart.

2. Use calcium-fortified soymilk in cream soups or stews that call for broth-based gravies.

3. Add canned salmon with the bones to a light tomato-based pasta sauce.

4. Slip extra calcium into cream-based soups and sauces by adding a few tablespoons of powdered milk to them.

5. Add nonfat milk, powdered milk, or yogurt to fruit smoothies.

6. Add 1 to 2 tablespoons of powdered milk to muffin, cake, and quick bread recipes.

7. Add 1 to 2 tablespoons of powdered milk to meat loaf, stuffing, and casseroles.

8. Cook oatmeal and other hot cereals with milk instead of water.

9. Use yogurt instead of milk on dry cereal.

10. Top hot cereal with frozen yogurt or low-fat frozen dairy-based dessert.

11. Add milk or yogurt to eggs before cooking an omelette or scrambling eggs.

12. While cooking eggs, throw in some calcium-rich tofu cubes.

13. Top your calcium-enriched omelette or eggs with low-fat cheese.

14. Throw a few dried figs into your lunch bag.

15. Top salads, pastas, and casseroles with almonds or hazelnuts.

16. Go for the cheese-filled pastas instead of meat-filled—like ricotta or gorgonzola ravioli.

17. Keep a bowl of almonds or hazelnuts available to replace other snacks.

18. Mix chopped almonds or hazelnuts into plain yogurt along with honey and fruit.

19. Sprinkle Parmesan cheese or Romano cheese on tossed salads.

20. Add calcium-fortified juice to muffin, pancake, or waffle recipes.

21. Eat sardines, either oil-based or in tomato sauce, with the bones.

22. Mix canned salmon with the bones into mayonnaise and seasonings for an appetizer spread or for your sandwich.

23. Serve diced, cooked kale or young collard, turnip, or mustard greens or broccoli on top of pasta.

24. Experiment with bok choy and other Chinese vegetables.

25. Puree calcium-set tofu in a blender or food processor with some ricotta or cottage cheese as a filling for lasagna or other pasta.

26. Use pureed calcium-set tofu as a replacement or for part of mayonnaise or sour cream in a dip or salad dressing.

27. Add shredded kale or greens to broth with some calcium-set tofu cubes.

28. Prepare eggs, pancakes, or waffles with milk (or try a yogurt-milk mix to give them a slight tang).

29. Drink calcium-fortified juice for breakfast or as a snack.

30. Add low-fat cheese to sandwiches or salads.

31. Sprinkle sugared almonds on top of cooked mustard greens or kale for a delicate contrast to the greens' tangy flavor.

32. Choose coleslaw or cabbage-based salads or soups.

33. Sprinkle Parmesan cheese or Romano cheese on garlic bread.

34. Include cooked collard or mustard greens with pasta.

35. Add small dices of calcium-set tofu to your meat-based stir-fries.

36. Top diced calcium-set tofu and pasta shells with a spicy pasta sauce and top with some cheese.

37. Stuff potatoes with broccoli and beans and low-fat cheese.

38. Add broccoli flowerets to salads or pastas.

39. Use pureed calcium-set tofu in place of evaporated milk in custards or pies (increase seasoning a bit).

40. Add snips of greens, pieces of broccoli, and some beans to soups and stews.

41. Use corn tortillas that have been made with calcium—top with beans, veggies, and some low-fat cheese.

42. Try tofu "croutons" (small tofu cubes) in green or fruit salads that are topped with your favorite dressing.

43. Top baked potatoes with yogurt.

44. Sprinkle chopped, toasted almonds on top of the yogurt on top of the potato.

45. Replace mayonnaise in fruit salads completely or at least by half with yogurt.

46. Sauté some kohlrabi in a small amount of olive oil with salt and Italian seasoning as a new side dish.

47. Sauté red cabbage with green apple and top with almonds.

48. Order a big dish of Chinese vegetables when you have Chinese food.

49. Combine soft goat cheese with crisp-cooked broccoli and sun-dried tomatoes with your favorite rice or pasta.

50. Drink flavored soymilk as a snack instead of juice or coffee.

Some Final Words

With some effort, you can help reduce the likelihood of having a calcium-deficient diet. Additionally, foods that are high in calcium power are also very well balanced naturally by other nutrients that help calcium perform some of the body's functions. Being familiar with the calcium power of different foods will help you choose calcium-rich foods without overindulging in high-calcium, high-fat foods.

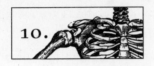

Understanding Calcium Supplements

∞

Nutrition experts overwhelmingly agree that the optimum way to maximize calcium's benefits is to get our calcium from calcium-rich foods and beverages. However, for many of us, adding calcium tablets to our daily routine may be a wise and practical choice. Dietary calcium intake has been found to be inadequate in virtually all age groups of Americans, and taking a regular calcium supplement will help to insure that we get adequate calcium each day. But there can be some drawbacks to taking a calcium supplement. Sometimes, when we rely on a supplement, we get a false sense of security and end up putting less effort into getting calcium from food. After all, it takes much less thought to swallow a tablet than to consciously make calcium-rich food choices. Also, although supplemental calcium increases our calcium intake, it doesn't provide a balanced mix of other important nutrients and compounds found in food. Many calcium-rich foods and beverages give us protein, vitamins, minerals, phytochemicals, fiber, and other nutrients that we may otherwise miss out on. We are unlikely to find a complete and balanced mix of nutritious compounds in a calcium tablet.

In general, calcium supplements should not be used to supplant calcium-rich foods, but to bolster calcium intake. So, while it may be an excellent idea for many of us to supplement our diets with calcium, we should still make certain that we eat a variety of calcium-rich foods and beverages every day, such as those discussed in the previous chapter.

Those Who May Benefit from Calcium Supplements

All healthy people who consume a wide variety of foods and have good appetites would benefit more if they got all of their calcium requirements from the foods they eat rather than relying on a calcium supplement. But there are special circumstances when it may be necessary for some people to take supplemental calcium in order for them to meet their calcium needs. For a reminder about how much calcium you should be getting, see Chapter 8.

Those with Limited Appetites

Women and men who are unable to consume enough calories to meet their needs might benefit from taking calcium supplements. These people may have little or no appetite or may be taking medications that interfere with regular eating. Unless they are able to eat two to three servings of yogurt or drink milk almost daily, in addition to eating other calcium-rich foods, it's unlikely that they will be able to get enough calcium to meet their bodies' needs.

Those with a Habitual Low Calcium Intake

Some people may think that they have well-balanced diets only to learn that they are not getting enough calcium every day. If you think you may be one of those people, try writing down everything you eat for three random nonconsecutive days during a typical week—use a non-work day as one of the days because eating habits typically change with a change in routine. Then, do a rough estimate of your calcium intake by checking what you ate against Table 9.1 on page 123.

If your calcium intake was low each day (600 milligrams or less of calcium), it may be a good idea to consider taking a calcium supplement. However, you should try adding more calcium-rich foods to your diet before turning to calcium tablets.

Those Who Cannot Tolerate Calcium-Rich Foods

There are special circumstances that make it difficult or impossible for some of us to get enough calcium. Adults and children who are lactose intolerant or who have milk allergies usually must avoid some or even all dairy foods, which are among calcium's richest food sources. (See Chapter 9 for more information on milk allergies and lactose intolerance.) Children who habitually eat a very limited number of foods, cannot drink milk, or reject other foods such as calcium-fortified orange juice, tofu, or leafy greens might also benefit from a calcium supplement—at least until they begin to eat a wider variety of foods, which generally happens with age. With children in particular, be sure to check with their pediatricians before giving them calcium supplements.

Those with Reduced Ability to Absorb Calcium

Finally, there are some groups of people, especially many of the elderly, who may not be able to absorb calcium very well. As a normal part of aging, stomach acid secretion usually decreases, which diminishes the efficiency of calcium absorption. (Calcium absorption is enhanced in an acidic environment.) In addition, calcium absorption may be reduced in part due to interactions with medications or a deficiency of vitamin D, a common condition in the elderly.

Those at Risk for Increased Bone Loss

The vast majority of menopausal and postmenopausal women have very low calcium intakes of about 600 milligrams a day in contrast to the recommendation of 1,000 milligrams a day for women on hormone replacement therapy and 1,500 milligrams per day for those not taking replacement hormones. Although calcium has its limits to how much it can do to prevent the loss of minerals from bone as we age, some health experts recommend that especially this group of women consider supplemental calcium to help slow the dramatic rate of bone loss that occurs with the decrease of hormone secretion. In studies involving menopausal and postmenopausal women who had taken calcium supplements, some found that the women did not lose bone and that some had even shown an increase in bone mass by about one percent per year. Other research has shown that a calcium supplement paired with hormone replacement therapy is even more beneficial than a calcium supplement alone. But don't forget, consuming enough calcium from food and regular weight-bearing activity continue to be very important for bone health. If there are no other reasons, medical or physiological, that rule out taking supplemental calcium, these groups of women should certainly discuss taking a calcium supplement with their health-care professional.

As men age, they are also at increased risk of bone loss, although not at such a great extent as women. The average intake of calcium for this group is about 700 to 800 milligrams per day, which is significantly lower than the current recommendation of 1,000 milligrams per day. If there are no other precluding reasons, they might also benefit from taking a calcium supplement and should consult their health-care professionals.

Those Who May Not Benefit from Calcium Supplements

Most of us wouldn't be adversely affected by taking in a reasonable amount of calcium in supplemental form on a daily basis. Combined dietary and supplemental calcium intake up to 2,500 milligrams per day is considered to be a safe upper limit for most people. (See Chapter 8 for recommended calcium intakes.) However, there are some people who should avoid taking calcium supplements under certain circumstances.

Those Who Are Taking Certain Prescription Medications

Anyone taking a medication on a regular basis should check with a health-care professional before taking calcium supplements. Long-term use of diuretics, also called "water pills," commonly prescribed for high blood pressure, congestive heart failure, and some other conditions, may cause blood calcium levels to rise. Diuretics can alter the way the kidneys excrete calcium, which may result in calcium toxicity, leading to kidney damage.

If you are taking calcium channel blockers or a beta-blocker— popular drugs prescribed for high blood pressure and other heart problems—your doctor may need to monitor or adjust the amount of the medication you take. Calcium supplementation may possibly modify the effectiveness of these drugs—although the extent of the effects is unknown.

Finally, the interactions between tetracycline-containing antibiotics, which are some of the most commonly prescribed drugs used to fight infections, and calcium are two-fold. When the antibiotic is taken within an hour of either taking a calcium supplement or eating calcium-containing food, it will bind with calcium, decreasing the amount that is absorbed and also decreasing the antibiotic's effectiveness. Tetracycline-containing antibiotics typically have a warning about this calcium interaction directly on the prescription bottle label. See Table 3.1 on page 31 for more information concerning calcium-medication interactions.

Those Who Are Taking Iron Supplements

Calcium from milk or supplements, in particular calcium carbonate, can decrease the amount of iron that is absorbed by the body by as much as half. (Supplements made from calcium citrate do not appear to have this effect.) To help counter this interference, iron supplements should be taken with meals and calcium supplements should be taken between meals. Sometimes calcium isn't as well absorbed when not taken with a meal. So, to help maximize calcium absorption, take it with a source of lactose and vitamin D, such as vitamin D-fortified milk.

Those Who Have a Family History of Kidney Stones

The myth that calcium causes kidney stones has been largely disproved. But if you have a family history of kidney stones, you may be at higher risk of having a recurrent episode. In some people with a previous history of kidney stones, a high calcium intake may increase the excretion of calcium through the urine, which might stimulate stone formation although more research is needed to confirm this. See Chapter 5 for more information concerning calcium and kidney stones.

The Dual-Approach Route to Calcium Intake

Using a calcium supplement to balance calcium intake from foods may be the best and most practical way to insure that we are taking in proper amounts of this essential mineral. A practical situation for a normal, healthy person whose dietary calcium intake is marginal would be to use calcium supplementation to bridge the calcium gap, while continuing each day to consume a variety of calcium-rich foods. Then, depending on how much dietary calcium is consumed, vary the amount taken in supplemental form. This really isn't as hard as it sounds. First, become familiar with the average calcium content in the calcium-rich foods and beverages you normally consume, and simply keep a mental note during the day whenever you take in a good source of calcium. This takes very little time. At dinner, review the amount of calcium you had that day and decide if it is necessary to take a calcium supplement depending on where your calcium estimate fell.

With this strategy, there are multiple benefits. Relying on food sources for calcium will lessen chances of a calcium toxicity from ingesting an excess amount of calcium. The intake of other nutrients and phytochemicals that accompany calcium in food will be enhanced, many of which, as we have learned, are needed for calcium to function optimally and to help provide protection against disease. In addition, the body appears to have built-in control mechanisms for how much calcium it will absorb. When there's too much calcium or not enough, it will adapt by modifying the amount that is absorbed according to what it needs. Casually taking calcium supplements over and above our needs could result in excess calcium being excreted from the body.

By using the "dual-approach" strategy, you will be more likely to remain centered on calcium-rich food sources as the ultimate way to get calcium. This strategy is a balanced and moderate method that will help you increase your dietary calcium intake, while boosting the power you will get from calcium. If you have questions about whether or not this dual approach is for you, talk to your health-care professional.

Piecing Together the Supplement Puzzle

The world of calcium supplements is like a puzzle, containing many pieces to be put together before you can appreciate the whole picture. Putting this puzzle together means sorting through some information. Fortunately, even with many pieces of information to consider, the vast majority of healthy people will effectively utilize most kinds of calcium supplements. Calcium supplements differ by the amount of elemental calcium (that is, the amount of actual calcium) they contain; by the number of tablets needed to get the desired amount of elemental calcium; with what they are chemically paired; and by how well the calcium is generally absorbed by the body. Calcium supplements also vary in the other kinds of nutrients or ingredients added intentionally or those which are naturally found in them.

Figure 10.1 on page 140 provides you with a comparison of the amount of elemental calcium in the principal forms of calcium supplements that are currently available. You can see that a supplement can contain as little as 10 percent to as much as 40 percent elemental calcium. Calcium carbonate contains the most elemental calcium per tablet. The amount of elemental calcium determines how many tablets you will need to take and how much it will cost you to get your recommended amount. The more elemental calcium in a product, the fewer tablets you need to take, and thus usually the less expensive it will be. Because calcium is so active, it is always chemically paired with another substance. The kinds of substances with which calcium is chemically partnered are also given in Figure 10.1. Furthermore, nearly all of these forms of supplemental calcium are absorbed by healthy adults almost equally and as well as calcium from foods. By only a few percentage points, calcium citrate malate has been shown to be the better absorbed than other calcium supplements.

Numerous "extras" may be added to supplemental calcium. To a large degree, added vitamins and minerals, such as magnesium and zinc, are not believed to be a necessary part of a calcium tablet. This is because if you take a supplement that already contains adequate amounts of the added nutrients, if you have a balanced diet, or if you regularly eat food fortified with these nutrients, you could be at risk for getting excess amounts of them. If you think you have an inadequate intake of the added nutrients, check with your health-care professional before opting for calcium tablets containing them. In addition, a new generation of calcium supplements is emerging that contain phytochemicals or other compounds with claims of added benefit to your bones or your health. At this time, more research is needed to confirm whether or not any of these compounds, such as phytoestrogens, are really of benefit. They may not be worth the premium price that usually accompanies them.

By sorting through these differences, pieces of the calcium supplement puzzle should fall into place. You'll have a better idea of which type of supplemental calcium is most suitable for your needs. Below are some of the unique characteristics of the most common forms of calcium supplements.

Calcium Carbonate

Calcium carbonate contains the most elemental calcium per tablet, and it is also the most commonly available of all the calcium supplements. It is well absorbed by the body and is usually the least expensive because so much more elemental calcium can be packed into a single tablet. By weight, about 40 percent of each tablet is elemental calcium. On average, it takes about two to three tablets to get 1,000 milligrams of calcium.

Some antacids that are promoted for their calcium content are made of calcium carbonate. Since calcium is best absorbed in an acidic environment, it may sound illogical for calcium to be contained in an antacid. Although naively taking too many antacids can be harmful, it is believed that by taking only what is needed to meet your recommended calcium intake, there is little risk of getting an excess amount of calcium. With some brands, only two to three antacid tablets will satisfy most people's recommended daily amount. Note, though, that some calcium-containing antacids may also contain magnesium and aluminum hydroxide, which can interfere with calcium retention by the body.

Moreover, using an antacid for supplemental calcium may not be beneficial for some people, especially older adults. This is because as we age, our stomachs produce less stomach acid when food is eaten, a condition called *atrophic gastritis,* which affects at least 20 percent of people over sixty years of age. With less stomach acid or when a calcium carbonate-containing antacid is taken by itself between meals, less of the elemental calcium may become available for absorption.

Calcium carbonate is better absorbed when taken with meals because of the presence of stomach acid, and also because the presence of food slows stomach emptying, allowing more time for the tablet to be broken down and the calcium to be absorbed. To enhance calcium absorption when supplementation occurs between meals, drink some milk (which contains vitamin D to help with absorption) or a glass of orange juice (which provides some acidity) with the calcium carbonate tablet.

In addition, there are anecdotal reports that calcium carbonate may cause bloating, stomach irritation, or constipation, although scientific documentation about these effects is lacking. If you experience these kinds of side effects with calcium carbonate, make sure you are drinking ample fluids, especially milk to help prevent or reduce the symptoms or switch to another form of calcium supplement. Also, if you are taking two to three tablets per day, spacing them out over the course of the day may help reduce the possibility of constipation and may help them be better absorbed.

Calcium Citrate

Of all the calcium supplement options, calcium citrate is one of the best-absorbed forms. It is absorbed efficiently when taken either with meals or between meals. But because of its large chemical structure, it's hard to fit a lot of elemental calcium into a tablet. Thus, you'll need to take more calcium citrate tablets than you would of some other kinds. To reach 1,000 milligrams per day, you may need to take twelve tablets each day.

You will also see the compound calcium citrate malate as the form contained in calcium-fortified juices and some other beverages. This is similar to calcium citrate, but currently is available only in certain brands of calcium-fortified beverages and supplements. Both calcium citrate and calcium citrate malate appear to be absorbed by the body at about the same rate.

Calcium Gluconate and Calcium Lactate

Both calcium gluconate and calcium lactate are absorbed efficiently by the body. But because they are similar to calcium citrate in the size of their chemical structure, it is hard to pack a lot of elemental calcium into calcium lactate or calcium gluconate tablets. Only about 20 percent of a calcium lactate tablet is elemental calcium, whereas in calcium gluconate only 9 percent is elemental calcium. More lactate and gluconate tablets will be needed to get the recommended amounts of calcium.

Calcium Phosphate

Calcium phosphate supplies more elemental calcium than calcium lactate or calcium gluconate, but is still less than the amount that we get from calcium carbonate. Calcium phosphate comes in different forms, such as calcium di-phosphate (or dibasic) and calcium tri-phosphate. Calcium di-phosphate is absorbed as well as most other supplements, while calcium tri-phosphate may be less well absorbed by some people.

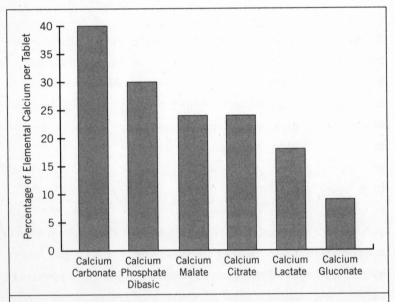

FIGURE 10.1. The percentage of elemental calcium contained in each tablet of different calcium supplements.

Calcium Chelates

Calcium chelates (pronounced *key-lates*) are among the newest and most expensive upscale version of calcium supplements. They are compounds of calcium that are combined with amino acids. The word chelate means claw, and in these supplements, one of the molecules is linked to the other in a claw-like manner. As a result, theoretically, the calcium is better absorbed. So far, it seems that absorption is improved only by a small amount, calling into question whether or not the much higher price is worth it.

The "Natural" Calcium Triad

Three popular "natural" calcium supplements are heavily promoted and widely available. While they can truthfully boast that they are natural, in this case, natural definitely isn't better. None of these forms of calcium is recommended.

Bone Meal This form of supplemental calcium contains natural bone meal and has a bad reputation that is well justified. Bone meal is made from fresh, degreased, and ground or crushed animal bones. It supplies calcium phosphate and other bone-related mineral elements in proper balance—which, considering the source, is no surprise. Unfortunately, the body does not absorb bone meal very well, and worse yet, some bone meal products have been found to contain large amounts of heavy metals, such as lead and other environmental pollutants, such as pesticide residues and plutonium.

All naturally derived sources of calcium contain some lead, because it is a pollutant that is widespread in our environment. However, in comparison to bone meal as well as dolomite and oyster shell calcium, which are discussed below, other kinds of calcium salts that are mined from the earth, like calcium carbonate, contain amounts of lead at levels that are in accordance with federal or state laws. Although only trace amounts of lead are found in other naturally de-rived forms of supplemental calcium, the amount of lead in bone meal can be extraordinarily high. This is because of lead's natural affinity to accumulate in bones. In one report, lead concentrations in a sample of bone meal supplements were up to forty times higher than that of calcium carbonate and twice as high as calcium supple-ments made from oyster shells.

Over a long period of time, lead in the bloodstream poisons the body by interfering with red blood cells, which then become unable to perform their crucial roles in the body. Lead also affects white blood cells, impairing their ability to fight infection, and adversely affects the brain's ability to function causing nervous system disor-ders and impairing mental health. Recently, lead has been linked to heart disease, high blood pressure, and kidney problems. Lead is par-ticularly risky for pregnant and nursing women and especially to children, who absorb five to ten times the amount of lead as adults. It stunts growth in children and can cause permanent behavioral problems and learning disabilities. Therefore, no one should take bone meal for his or her source of supplemental calcium, especially not children or pregnant or nursing women.

The good news is that the higher your intake of calcium, the less likely that you will experience adverse effects from lead. This is be-cause lead that has built up in the bones becomes a health problem only when too much is released into the blood, which happens whenever too much calcium is withdrawn from the bones; that is, when calcium intake is low. In addition, calcium has been shown to limit the absorption of lead, which provides some added built-in protection.

Dolomite Often sold as a "calcium-magnesium" supplement, dolomite is composed of calcium magnesium carbonate that has been mined from the earth's crust. It's the same compound found in marble and limestone. By virtue of being within the earth, dolomite accumulates trace elements and heavy metals, such as mercury, arsenic, and lead. Similar to bone meal, there are similar kinds of problems with dolomite due to the potential contamination by heavy metals. In addition, it is not well absorbed and has been found to interfere with absorption of other minerals. As such, this form of supplemental calcium also should be avoided.

Oyster Shell Calcium Supplemental calcium derived from ground oyster shells is comprised of calcium carbonate, but this calcium carbonate is poorly absorbed by the body. Oyster shell calcium may be mined from fossilized sources, and like dolomite, may be contaminated by heavy metals that have built up over the years. A comparison of seventy different calcium-supplement products showed a considerable amount of lead as well as aluminum contamination in commonly available oyster shell brands. It also should be avoided.

Getting the Most from Your Calcium Supplement

Deciding on the form of supplemental calcium that you want based on your preferences doesn't automatically insure that you will get the most benefit from it. There are additional pieces to the supplement puzzle that must be considered. For example, the amount of benefit will be determined partly by your ability to take and remember to take your supplement. How well your calcium tablet is absorbed may depend on when you take your tablet or the manufacturer's technique used to make the tablets. Below are some additional tips.

Take a Form That Works for You

There are several different ways to get your supplemental calcium. You can take it as a tablet that you swallow, chew, or dissolve in your mouth; as a powdered preparation that you mix with a liquid; or even in ready-to-take liquid form. Choose the form of calcium supplement that you will be able to take and will remember to take. If you have difficulty swallowing tablets, consider a liquid or one that dissolves in your mouth. If you need convenience, a powdered preparation that requires mixing may not work for you.

Schedule the Best Supplement-Taking Time

To get the benefit of a calcium supplement, it needs to be taken regularly. Because any new routine takes time to get used to, be sure to choose a time for supplement taking that you are most likely to remember. Many people find that linking supplement taking with routine daily tasks helps them to remember. For example, take a supplement with the morning meal and then with the evening meal. Or, if you work, keep some at the office and take them during your break or at lunch.

Also, as mentioned previously, calcium absorption by the body is determined in part by its needs. The more the body needs, the more it will absorb; the less it needs, the less it will absorb. Overloading your digestive system with too much supplemental calcium at one time may result in loss of calcium and your money. The body may not be able to absorb very large doses all at once. So, it would seem preferable to take your calcium in divided doses, particularly if you are taking more than 500 milligrams per day. The calcium will probably be better absorbed if you space your doses apart—like at breakfast and at dinner. It really comes back down to the principals of moderation and balance. But if you are only able to take your supplement once a day, losing a little extra calcium is better than not taking any at all.

Take with Food to Enhance Absorption

Taking a calcium supplement with food enhances calcium absorption. Stomach acid secretion increases when we eat, which increases intestinal acidity. Food may also slow down calcium's travel time through the intestinal tract, and the digestive action may help break down the tablet, giving it a better chance to be absorbed by the body.

Take Into Account What Else You're Taking

If you take a supplement that contains iron, take it at a time different from when you take your calcium supplement. Calcium changes the acidic environment of the stomach in such a way that it interferes with iron absorption. But don't be concerned if you are taking a multivitamin and mineral tablet that includes both of these minerals. Usually, there's only 100 to 200 milligrams of calcium in a multivitamin and mineral tablet, which won't cause a problem with iron absorption.

Likewise, be sure to check with your doctor or pharmacist if you are taking any medications or other nutritional supplements that could interact with calcium. See Table 3.1 on page 31 for more information about calcium and medication interactions.

Insure Tablet Reliability

Some calcium supplements have been found to be highly unabsorbable by the body due to the manufacturing technique used to make the tablets. Some types of processing makes it difficult for the stomach acid to penetrate the tablet so that it can dissolve. Such a calcium supplement will do you no good if it passes through your digestive tract intact. Unfortunately, not all tablets are tested for how well they dissolve once they have reached the stomach. So, it is not always clear how efficiently each of them will be absorbed by the body. If a supplement label lists the letters "USP," which stands for the United States Pharmacopeia (an independent scientific organization), this means it meets strict standards for dissolution. But, if you want to test the ability of your calcium tablet to dissolve in the stomach, drop the tablet in three-quarters of a cup of vinegar and stir every five minutes for thirty minutes. A high quality tablet will dissolve within that time.

Minimize Potential Side Effects

Some people have reported experiencing constipation, bloating, and/or excess gas from some types of calcium supplements. If this occurs, be sure that you are getting enough fiber in your diet and that you are drinking ample fluid every day—at least one to two quarts of any liquid that does not contain caffeine or alcohol, such as water, juice, or milk—and try splitting up tablet taking into at least two different dosages during the day.

Watch Out for Supplement Hype and Higher Cost

Ignore eye-catching labels and glamorous claims. Whenever you see the word "natural" or "organic" on a supplement, think twice before you pay extra. On calcium supplement labels, these claims have no legal meaning—in contrast to labels on organic vegetables and other foods, which do have specific legal meanings. The same is true for claims such as "no sugar," "no starch," or "no preservatives." These are legally devoid of meaning relative to the calcium supplement itself. They are typical marketing strategies aimed at getting you to buy the product. Also, it's best to avoid products that make "high potency" claims. More is not necessarily better, and as discussed in Chapter 8, too much calcium can accumulate and cause health problems.

Some calcium supplements cost more than others. Calcium carbonate is usually among the least expensive and yields the highest amount of elemental calcium and best absorbability for the number of tablets needed. A generic brand of calcium carbonate without added ingredients will work just as well as a major brand with hyperbolic claims in a more attractive bottle.

Some Final Words

Taking a calcium supplement may be an important option for some groups of people, since it is better to take supplemental calcium than to have a calcium-deficient diet. But supplements will usually be poor second choices to calcium-rich foods. If you choose to supplement your diet with a calcium tablet, do so to complement your intake of calcium-rich foods, not to replace it. When you are considering the use of a supplement, be sure to think about the form of the supplement and the schedule that's most suitable for you. And always check with your health-care professional to see if supplements are right for you. Taking a few minutes to put together the pieces of the calcium-supplement puzzle will help you to maximize calcium's many benefits.

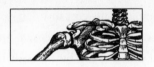

Conclusion

THERE is no doubt that we know more today about the importance of calcium than ever before. The achievements of science and medicine have given us extraordinary means of bringing to light calcium's life-sustaining roles and the ability to delve into the uncharted waters of calcium and its links to health and protection from disease. The escalating interest and excitement generated by calcium is only in its infancy. We have much to learn in our quest for answers to its mysteries. Future examination of the benefits of calcium will likely continue to yield surprising health-giving results, further emphasizing our need for an ample supply of calcium day in and day out.

There is no doubt that many of the changes of our modern times are working against calcium, hampering its ability to perform as optimally as it potentially could. We are doing much less bone-strengthening physical activity than our grandparents did, and because physical activity is central to bone health, this may also influence the way that calcium works in our bodies. Unfortunately, we are getting much less calcium from our diets than our ancestors did, and some foods we eat have been so processed that little of their original nutrition remains. Calcium-robbing meats and other non-dairy animal foods have too much plate space in many of our diets. Also, we have so many medications, often crucial to our health, which may affect calcium functioning. Finally, many of us spend too little time in sunlight, which our bodies need to synthesize vitamin D—a vitamin that plays a crucial role in calcium absorption.

There are three key concepts that you have learned in this book that you should always remember. The first is that calcium has many roles in the body that bring vigor and vitality to life, which extend far beyond that of just building bones and teeth. Second, the degree of calcium's many benefits depends on other components of food, on physical activity, on sunlight, and on other factors in our lifestyles and backgrounds. And third, calcium is a very active mineral; our bones are living tissues that are constantly being dismantled and re-built from the time we are conceived until the time we die. Bones are the body's almost endless supply of calcium. This reservoir provides the blood with calcium, which enables crucial metabolic activities to take place.

Some of the key benefits of calcium include the following:

- Calcium is a cornerstone mineral of our bones and teeth and a crucial mineral in our blood.
- Calcium keeps us from bleeding uncontrollably, it keeps our muscles and nerves in action, and it helps to keep our cells functioning properly.
- Calcium is gaining a presence as an important player in helping to protect us from many chronic diseases, such as hypertension, colon cancer, kidney stones, and even possibly premenstrual syndrome and breast cancer.

There are four key steps in proper calcium nutrition. If you follow these steps, you'll be sure to get the amount of calcium that your body requires to function at optimal levels.

1. Consume an ample amount of calcium-rich foods every day, including fermented milks, such as yogurt, and other milk products; green vegetables, such as broccoli and kale; nuts, such as almonds and hazelnuts; and cooked dry beans. If the centerpiece of your meals is animal-based, find alternative choices that are high in calcium power.

2. If getting enough calcium every day is not possible, consider taking a good calcium supplement. Take more or less depending on the rest of your diet.

3. Remember that calcium, or any other nutrient for that matter, does not function in isolation. There are many interactions among substances found in foods; it's important to think of calcium in terms of your overall eating pattern.

4. Be sure to do some bone-strengthening exercise every day. The human body was made to be physically active. Many of our bodily functions work best when we are active on a regular basis—the heart is helped, the muscles are worked, the blood flows better, and our digestive systems work better.

The power of calcium has been appreciated since ancient times. Its vital roles in sustaining life must be respected. But it also must be remembered that calcium works as part of a team that keeps the human body working at its best. The ultimate key to unlocking the power of calcium is moderation and balance in all things. To the extent that calcium is an integral part of our daily lives, we will be helping to ensure that we and our children can enjoy the greatest gift life has to offer: good health. Remember, the human body needs the power of calcium day in and day out.

Glossary

Blood calcium. The 1 to 2 percent of the body's total calcium that is found in the blood. Blood calcium is essential to numerous vital bodily functions, such as blood clotting and muscle contraction.

Bone density. The amount of bone mass.

Bone mass. The actual amount of bone-related minerals in the bones.

Bone mineralization. The process by which the principal bone-related minerals (calcium, phosphorus, magnesium, and zinc) harden on the protein matrix of a growing bone to provide skeletal strength.

Bone remodeling. The dynamic process of breaking down and rebuilding bone to replace old bone with new tissue; occurs continuously throughout life.

Calcitonin. A hormone produced by the thyroid gland that helps to lower blood calcium by reducing the amount of calcium that is withdrawn from bone.

Calcium. A moderately hard, silver-white metallic mineral that is essential for life.

Collagen. The major supportive protein component on which bone-related minerals are deposited.

Enzymes. Proteins secreted by the body that promote or accelerate biochemical reactions in the body.

Estrogen. Female hormone that helps build and maintain bone.

Fracture. A crack or break in a bone.

Hormone. Chemical messengers produced by the body and secreted by a variety of glands in response to altered conditions in the body.

Hydroxyapatite. Calcium-containing mineral crystals of bone.

Lactose intolerance. A condition that results in the limited or complete inability to break down milk sugar, so that it can be absorbed into the bloodstream.

Metabolism. All of the chemical processes and reactions that take place in living cells.

Osteoporosis. Loss of bone minerals, resulting in porous, weakened, and fragile bones that are easily susceptible to fracture.

Parathyroid hormone (PTH). A hormone produced by the body that is crucial for regulating levels of calcium in the blood through its effects on bone and kidney; promotes the release of calcium from bone.

Peak bone mass. The highest attainable bone mass, developed during the first three decades of life.

Phytochemicals. A general term for hundreds of compounds found only in unrefined plant foods with protective biological activity.

Progesterone. Female hormone that helps build and maintain bone.

Saturated fat. The predominant type of fat found in whole milk and low-fat dairy foods, beef, pork, lamb, veal, poultry, and hydrogenated vegetable oils. Of all dietary fat, it is the strongest contributor to the elevation of blood cholesterol levels, which is associated with an increased risk of heart disease.

Testosterone. The principal male hormone that is important for maintaining muscle mass and bone tissue.

Unsaturated fat. The predominant type of fat found in many plant foods, such as nuts and seeds, as well as oily fish, such as salmon; associated with lowering blood cholesterol levels, which is linked to a reduced risk of heart disease.

Vertebrae. Segments of bones that make up the spinal column; back bones.

Weight-bearing exercise. Physical activity, such as walking, running, hiking, tennis, and heavy gardening or housework, that helps to maintain bone density.

Additional Resources

✌

Books containing calcium-rich recipes and/or more information about wholesome eating:

Cole, Candia Lea. *Not Milk . . . NUT MILKS!* Santa Barbara, CA: Woodbridge Press, 1990.

Katzen, Mollie. *Vegetable Heaven*. New York, NY: Hyperion, 1997.

Lappé, Frances Moore. *Diet for a Small Planet*. New York, NY: Ballantine Books, 1982.

Margen, S. and Editors of the University of California at Berkeley Wellness Letter. *The Wellness Encyclopedia of Food and Nutrition: How to Buy, Store, and Prepare Every Fresh Food*. New York, NY: Random House, 1992.

Robertson, Laurel, Carol Flinders, and Brian Ruppenthal. *The New Laurel's Kitchen*. Berkeley, CA: Ten Speed Press, 1986.

Sass, Lorna. *Recipes from an Ecological Kitchen*. New York, NY: Morrow, 1992.

Spiller, Gene and Bonnie Bruce. *The Cancer Survivor's Nutrition and Health Guide.* Rocklin, CA: Prima Publishing, 1997.

Spiller, Gene and Rowena Hubbard. *Nutrition Secrets of the Ancients.* Rocklin, CA: Prima Publishing, 1996.

Spiller, Gene. *Eat Your Way to Better Health.* Rocklin, CA: Prima Publishing, 1996.

Spiller, Gene. *Healthy Nuts.* New York, NY: Avery, 2000.

Tatro, D. S. (ed.) *Drug Interaction Facts,* 5th ed. St. Louis, MO: A Wolters Kluwe Co, 1996.

Government and private resources for additional information: *(Addresses and telephone numbers are subject to change.)*

Food and Nutrition Information Center
USDA/National Agricultural Library, Room 304
10301 Baltimore Blvd.
Beltsville, MD 20705-2351
(301) 504–5719
Internet address: fnic@nalusda.gov

International Food Information Council (IFIC)
1100 Connecticut Avenue, NW, Suite 30
Washington, DC 20036
(202) 296–6540
Internet address: http://ificinfo.health.org

National Academy of Sciences/Food and Nutrition Board
2101 Constitution Avenue, NW
Washington, DC 20418
(202) 334–1732

National Center for Nutrition and Dietetics (NCND)
The American Dietetic Association
216 W Jackson Blvd, Suite 800
(312) 899–0040
General nutrition information: ext. 4653
Consumer nutrition hotline: (800) 366–1655
Internet address: www.eatright.org

National Dairy Council
10255 W Higgins Road, Suite 900
Rosemont, IL 60018-5616
(847) 803–2000
Internet address: www.nationaldairycouncil.org

National Institutes of Health
9000 Rockville Pike
Bethesda, MD 20892
(301) 496–4000
Internet address: http://www.osteo.org/osteo.html

National Osteoporosis Foundation
1150 17th Street, NW, Suite 500
Washington, DC 20036-4603
(800) 223–2226
Internet address: www.nof.org

National Yogurt Association
2000 Corporate Ridge
McLean, VA 22102
(703) 821–0770

Nutrition newsletters that provide an array of general nutrition and health information *(addresses and telephone numbers are subject to change):*

Consumer Reports on Health
Box 52148
Boulder, CO 80322-52148
(800) 234–2188

Environmental Nutrition
523 Riverside Dr., Suite 15-A
New York, NY 10024-6599

Mayo Clinic Health Letter
Subscription Services
PO Box 53889
Boulder, CO 80322-3889
(800) 333–9037

Tufts University Diet and Nutrition Letter
P.O. Box 57857
Boulder, CO 80322-3889
(800) 275–7581

University of California at Berkeley Wellness Letter
Health Letter Associates
P.O. Box 420148
Palm Coast, FL 32142
(800) 829–9080

References

⚛

Chapter 1: Calcium and Its History

Bogert, L. J., G. M. Briggs, and D. H. Calloway. *Nutrition and Physical Fitness*. Philadelphia: WB Saunders Co., 1973.

Encyclopaedia Britannica Inc. *The New Encyclopaedia Britannica*, vol. 2. Chicago: Encyclopaedia Britannica Inc., 1997.

Scala, J. *Making the Vitamin Connection: The Food Supplement Story*. New York: Harper and Row, 1985.

Spallholz, J. E., L. M. Boylan, and J. A. Driskell. *Nutrition: Chemistry and Biology*, 2nd ed. Boca Raton: CRC Press, 1999.

Chapter 2: Calcium's Metabolic Functions

Allen, L.H. and R.J.Wood. "Calcium and Phosphorus" in M. E. Shils, J. A. Olson, and M. Shike, (ed): *Modern Nutrition in Health and Disease*, 8th ed. Philadelphia: Lea and Febiger, 1994, pp 144–163.

Devlin, T. M. *Textbook of Biochemistry: With Clinical Correlations*, 3d ed. New York: Wiley-Liss, Inc., 1993.

Lobaugh, B. "Blood Calcium and Phosphorus Regulation." In J. B. Anderson and S. C. Garner (ed): *Calcium and Phosphorus in Health and Disease*. Boca Raton: CRC Press, 1996, pp 27–44.

Louie, D. "Intestinal Bioavailability and Absorption of Calcium." In J. B. Anderson and S. C. Garner (ed): *Calcium and Phosphorus in Health and Disease*. Boca Raton: CRC Press, 1996, pp 45–62.

Petersen, O.H., C.C.H. Petersen, and H. Kasai. "Calcium and hormone action." *Annual Reviews of Physiology* 56: 771, 1994.

Spallholz, J. E., L. M. Boylan, and J. A. Driskell. *Nutrition: Chemistry and Biology,* 2d ed. Boca Raton: CRC Press, 1999.

Vander, A. J., J. H. Sherman, and D. S. Luciano. *Human Physiology: The Mechanisms of Body Function*. New York: McGraw-Hill Book Co., 1970.

Chapter 3: The Formation and Maintenance of Bones and Teeth

Abrams, S. A. and J. E. Stuff. "Calcium metabolism in girls: current dietary intakes lead to low rates of calcium absorption and retention during puberty." *American Journal of Clinical Nutrition* 60: 739, 1994.

American Dietetic Association. "Position of the ADA: the impact of fluoride on dental health." *Journal of the American Dietetic Association* 94: 1428, 1994.

Anderson, J. B. "Dietary calcium and bone mass through the lifecycle." *Nutrition Today,* 25: 9, 1990.

DePaola, D., M. P. Faine, and R. I. Vogel. "Nutrition in Relation to Dental Medicine." In M. E. Shils, J. A. Olson, and M. Shike (ed): *Modern Nutrition in Health and Disease,* 8th ed. Philadelphia: Lea and Febiger, 1994, pp 1007–1028.

Felson, D. T., et al. "Alcohol intake and bone mineral density in older men and women: the Framingham study." *American Journal of Epidemiology* 142: 485, 1995.

Garner, S. C., J. B. Anderson, and W. Ambrose. "Skeletal Tissues and Mineralization." In J.B. Anderson and S.C. Garner, (ed): *Calcium and Phosphorus in Health and Disease.* Boca Raton: CRC Press, 1996, pp 97–118.

Green, J. "The Physiochemical Structure of Bone: Cellular and Noncellular Elements." *Mineral and Electrolyte Metabolism* 20: 7, 1994.

Holbrook, T. and E. Barrett-Connor. "A prospective study of alcohol consumption and bone mineral density." *British Medical Journal* 306: 1506, 1993.

Hopper, J. and E. Seeman. "The bone density of female twins discordant for tobacco use." *The New England Journal of Medicine* 330: 387, 1994.

Howat, P. M., et al. "The influence of diet, body fat, menstrual cycling and activity upon the bone density of females." *Journal of the American Dietetic Association* 89: 1305, 1989.

Jacob, S. W. *Structure and Function in Man,* 3rd ed. Philadelphia: W. B. Saunders, 1974.

Johnston, C., et al. "Calcium supplementation and increases in bone mineral density in children." *The New England Journal of Medicine* 327: 82, 1992.

Pocock, N. A., et al. "Genetic determinants of bone mass in adults: a twin study." *Journal of Clinical Investigation* 80: 706, 1987.

Pollitzer, W. S., and J.J.B. Anderson. "Ethnic and genetic differences in bone mass: a review with an hereditary vs. environmental perspective." *American Journal of Clinical Nutrition* 50:1244, 1989.

Seeman, E., et al. "Reduced bone mass in daughters of women with osteoporosis." *The New England Journal of Medicine* 320: 554, 1989.

Slemenda, C. "Cigarettes and the skeleton." *The New England Journal of Medicine* 323: 921, 1990.

Steinhausen, H. C. "The Course and Outcome of Anorexia Nervosa." In K. D. Brownell and C. G. Fairburn (ed): *Eating Disorders and Obesity: A Comprehensive Handbook.* London: Guilford Press, 1995, pp 234–127.

Tatro, D. S. (ed.). *Drug Interaction Facts,* 5th ed. St Louis, MO: A Wolters Kluwe Co, 1996.

Tilton, F.E., J.J.C. Degioanni, and V.S. Schneider. "Long-term Follow Up of Skylab Bone Demineralization." *Aviation, Space and Environmental Medicine* 51: 1209, 1980.

Vander, A. J., J.H. Sherman, and D. S. Luciano. *Human Physiology: The Mechanisms of Body Function.* New York: McGraw-Hill Book Co., 1970.

Whedon, G. D. "Changes in weightlessness in calcium metabolism and in the musculoskeletal system." *Physiologist* 25 (Suppl): S41, 1982.

Yaeger, K. K., et al. "The female athlete triad: disordered eating, amenorrhea, osteoporosis." *Medicine and Science in Sports and Exercise* 25: 775, 1993.

Chapter 4: Calcium's Connection to Osteoporosis

Arnauld, C. D., and S. D. Sanchez. "The role of calcium in osteoporosis." *Annual Reviews of Nutrition* 10: 397, 1990.

Bales, C. W. and J. B. Anderson. "Influence of Nutritional Factors On Bone Health In The Elderly." In J. B. Anderson and S. C. Garner, (ed): *Calcium and Phosphorus in Health and Disease.* Boca Raton: CRC Press. 1996, pp 319–340.

Cummings, S. R., et al.; "Epidemiology of osteoporosis and osteoporotic fractures." *Epidemiological Reviews* 7: 178, 1985.

Eastell, R. "Treatment of postmenopausal osteoporosis." *The New England Journal of Medicine* 338: 736, 1998.

Heaney, P. H. "Nutrition and Risk of Osteoporosis." In R. Marcus, D. Feldman, and J. Kelsey (ed): *Osteoporosis.* San Diego: Academic Press, 1996, pp 483–509.

Heaney, R. P. "Nutritional factors in osteoporosis." *Annual Reviews of Nutrition* 13: 287, 1993.

NIH Consensus Conference Panel. "NIH Consensus Conference: Osteoporosis." *Journal of the American Medical Association* 252: 799, 1984.

Recker, R. R., et al. "Change in Bone Mass Immediately Before Menopause." *Journal of Bone Mineral Research* 7: 857, 1992.

Riggs, B. L. and L. J. Melton. "Involutional osteoporosis." *The New England Journal of Medicine* 314:676, 1986.

Chapter 5: *The New Health Benefits of Calcium*

Alberts, D. S., et al. "Randomized, double-blinded, placebo-controlled study of effect of wheat bran fiber and calcium on fecal bile acids in patients with resected adenomatous colon polyps." *Journal of the National Cancer Institute* 88: 81, 1996.

Appel, L. J., et al. "A Clinical Trial of the Effects of Dietary Patterns on Blood Pressure." *The New England Journal of Medicine* 336: 1117, 1997.

Bostick, R. M., et al. "Relation of calcium, vitamin d, and dairy food intake to incidence of colon cancer among older women: the iowa women's health study." *American Journal of Epidemiology* 137: 1302, 1993.

Curhan, G. C., et al. "Comparison of dietary calcium with supplemental calcium and other nutrients as factors affecting the risk for kidney stones in women." *Annals of Internal Medicine* 126:497, 1997.

Favero, A., M. Parpinel, and S. Franceschi. "Diet and risk of breast cancer and major findings from an italian case-control study." *Biomedical Pharmacotherapy* 52: 109, 1998.

Hamet, P. "Evaluation of the scientific evidence for a relationship between calcium and hypertension." *Journal of Nutrition* 125 (Suppl): 311, 1995.

Jensen, O. M. and R. Maclennan. "Dietary factors and colorectal cancer in Scandinavia." *Israel Journal of Medical Science* 15: 329, 1979.

Kohlmeier, M., J. Saupe, and M. J. Shearer. "Risk of bone fracture in hemodialysis patients is related to vitamin k status." *Journal of Bone Mineral Research* 10: 5361, 1995.

Lipkin, M. "Calcium and breast cancer." *Journal of the American College of Nutrition* (Abstract) 17:503, 1998 (Abstr).

McCarron, D. A. and D. Hatton. "Dietary calcium and lower blood pressure: we can all benefit." *Journal of the American Medical Association* 275(editorial): 1128, 1996.

McCarron, D. A., C. D. Morris, and C. Cole. "Dietary calcium in human hypertension." *Science* 217: 267, 1982.

National Research Council (U.S.) Committee on Diet and Health. *Diet and Health: Implications for Reducing Chronic Disease Risk.* Washington, DC: National Academy of Sciences, 1989.

Osborne, C. G., et al. "Evidence for the relationship of calcium to blood pressure." *Nutrition Reviews* 54: 365, 1996.

Simon, J. A., et al. "Calcium intake and blood pressure in elderly women." *American Journal of Epidemiology* 31: 265, 1992.

Thys-Jacobs, S., et al. "Calcium carbonate and the premenstrual syndrome: Effects on premenstrual and menstrual symptoms. Premenstrual syndrome study group." *Obstetrics and Gynecology* 179: 444, 1998.

Chapter 6: Calcium's Interaction with Other Nutrients and Dietary Compounds

Allen, L. H., and R. J. Wood. "Calcium and Phosphorus." In M. E. Shils, J. A. Olson, and M. Shike (ed): *Modern Nutrition in Health and Disease,* 8th ed. Philadelphia: Lea and Febiger, 1994, pp 144–163.

Holick, M.F. "Vitamin D." In M. E. Shils, J. A. Olson, and M. Shike (ed): *Modern Nutrition in Health and Disease,* 8th ed. Philadelphia: Lea and Febiger, 1994, pp 308–325.

Marie, P. J., et al. "Histological osteomalacia due to dietary calcium deficiency in children." *The New England Journal of Medicine* 307: 584, 1982.

Olson, R. E. "Vitamin K." In M. E. Shils, J. A. Olson, and M. Shike (ed): *Modern Nutrition in Health and Disease,* 8th ed. Philadelphia: Lea and Febiger, 1994, pp 342–358.

Spallholz, J.E., L. M. Boylan, and J. A. Driskell. *Nutrition: Chemistry and Biology,* 2d ed. Boca Raton: CRC Press, 1999.

Chapter 7: Factors in Calcium Absorption

Andersson, H., B. Navert, S. A. Bingham, H. N. Englyst, and J. H. Cummings. "The effects of breads containing similar amounts of phytate but different amounts of wheat bran on calcium, zinc, and iron balance in man." *British Journal of Nutrition* 50: 503, 1983.

Anderson, J.J.B. and S. C. Garner. "Dietary Issues of Calcium and Phosphorus." In J. B. Anderson and S. C. Garner (ed): *Calcium and Phosphorus in Health and Disease.* Boca Raton: CRC Press, 1996, pp 7–26.

Berner, Y. N. and M. Shike. "Consequences of phosphate imbalance." *Annual Review of Nutrition* 8: 121, 1988.

Council on Scientific Affairs. "Dietary Fiber and Health." *Journal of the American Medical Association* 262: 542, 1989.

Eaton, S. B. and D. A. Nelson. "Calcium in evolutionary perspective." *American Journal of Clinical Nutrition* 54 (Suppl.): S281, 1991.

Gonick, H. C., G. Goldberg, and D. Mulcare. "Reexamination of the acid-ash content of several diets." *American Journal of Clinical Nutrition* 21: 898, 1968.

Harris, S. S. and B. Dawson-Hughes. "Caffeine and bone loss in healthy postmenopausal women." *American Journal of Clinical Nutrition* 60: 573, 1994.

Heaney, R. P. and C. M. Weaver. "Oxalate: effect on calcium absorbability." *American Journal of Clinical Nutrition* 50: 830, 1989.

Heaney, R. P., et al. "Absorbability of calcium from brassica vegetables." *Journal of Food Science* 58: 1378, 1993.

Heaney, R. P., C. M. Weaver, and R. R. Recker. "Calcium absorbability from spinach." *American Journal of Clinical Nutrition* 47: 707, 1988.

Heaney, R. P. "Protein intake and the calcium economy." *Journal of the American Dietetic Association* 3: 1259, 1993.

Jensen, O. M. and R. Maclennan. "Dietary factors and colorectal cancer in scandinavia." *Israel Journal of Medical Science* 15:329, 1979.

Kerstetter, J. E. and L. H. Allen "Dietary protein increases urinary calcium." *Journal of Nutrition* 120: 134, 1990.

Linkswiler, H. M., et al. "Protein-induced hypercalciuria." *Federal Proceedings* 40: 2429, 1981.

Linkswiler, H. M., C. L. Joyce, and C. R. Anand. "Calcium retention of young adult males as affected by level of protein and calcium intake." *Transactions of the New York Academy of Sciences* 36: 333, 1974.

Massey, L. and S. Whiting. "Caffeine, urinary calcium, calcium metabolism and bone." *Journal of Nutrition* 123: 1611, 1993.

McCance, R. A., E. M. Widdowson, and H. Lehmann. "The effect of protein intake on the absorption of calcium and magnesium." *Biochemistry Journal* 36: 686, 1942.

McCollum, E. V. and N. Simmonds. *The Newer Knowledge of Nutrition,* 3rd ed. New York: The MacMillan Company, 1925.

National Research Council. *Recommended Dietary Allowances,* 10th ed. Washington DC: National Academy Press, 1989.

Pennington, J.A.T. *Bowes and Church's Food Values of Portions Commonly Used,* 15th ed. New York: Harper Collins, 1989.

Schuette, S. A. and H. M. Linkswiler. "Effects on Ca and P metabolism by adding meat, meat plus milk, or purified proteins plus CA and P to a low protein diet." *Journal of Nutrition* 112: 338, 1982.

Spallholz, J. E., L. M. Boylan, and J. A. Driskell. *Nutrition: Chemistry and Biology,* 2d ed. Boca Raton: CRC Press, 1999.

Spencer, H. L., L. Kramer, and D. Osis. "Do protein and phosphorus cause calcium loss?" *Journal of Nutrition* 118: 657, 1988.

Spiller, G. A. (ed). *Dietary Fiber in Human Nutrition,* 2d ed. Boca Raton: CRC Press, 1993.

Tatro, D. S. (ed). *Drug Interaction Facts,* 5th ed. St Louis: A Wolters Kluwe Co., 1996.

Weaver, C. M., et al. "Human calcium absorption from whole wheat products." *Journal of Nutrition* 121: 1769, 1991.

Chapter 8: Getting Calcium in the Right Amounts

Alamo, K., et al. "Dietary intake of vitamins, minerals, and fiber of persons ages 2 months and over in the United States: third national health and nutrition examination survey, Phase 1, 1988–91." *Vital Health Statistics* No. 258, 1994.

Committee on Dietary Reference Intakes. *Dietary Reference Intakes for Calcium, Phosphorus, Magnesium, Vitamin D, and Fluoride.* Washington, DC: National Academy Press, 1997.

Fleming, K. H. and J. T. Heimbach. "Consumption of calcium in the U.S.: food sources and intake levels." *Journal of Nutrition* 124 (Suppl.): 1426S, 1994.

National Research Council. *Recommended Dietary Allowances,* 10th ed. Washington, DC: National Academy Press, 1989.

NIH Consensus Development Panel. "Optimal Calcium Intake." *Journal of the American Medical Association* 272: 1942, 1994.

Ramazzotto, L. T., et al. "Calcium nutrition and the aging process: a review." *Gerontology* 5: 159, 1986.

Riggs, B. L., et al. "Dietary calcium intake and rates of bone loss in women." *Journal of Clinical Investigation* 80: 979, 1987.

Chapter 9: Food Sources of Calcium

Block, G., C. M. Dresser, A. M. Harman, and M. D. Carroll. "Nutrient sources in the American diet: quantitative data from the NHANES II survey. Vitamins and minerals." *American Journal of Epidemiology* 122:13, 1985.

Eaton, S. B., M. Shostak, and M. Konner. *The Paleolithic Prescription.* New York: Harper & Row Publishers, 1988.

Ensminger, A. H., M. E. Ensminger, J. E. Konlande, and J.R.K. Robson. *The Concise Encyclopedia of Foods and Nutrition.* Boca Raton: CRC Press, 1995.

Flatz, C. "Genetics of Lactose Digestion in Humans." In H. Harris, K. Hirschhorn, and C. Flatz (ed). *Advances in Human Genetics.* New York: Plenum Press, 1987, pp 1–77.

Herbst, S. T. *The New Food Lover's Companion,* 2d ed. New York: Barron's Educational Series, Inc., 1995.

Hertzler, S. R., B. L. Huynh, and D. A. Savaiano. "How much lactose is low lactose?" *Journal of the American Dietetic Association* 96: 243, 1996.

Imagine Foods, Inc., Palo Alto, CA 94306.

McGee, H. *On Food and Cooking: The Science and Lore of the Kitchen.* NewYork: Charles Scribner's Sons, 1984.

Pennington, J.A.T. *Bowes and Church's Food Values of Portions Commonly Used,* 15th ed. New York: Harper Collins, 1989.

Saavedra, J. M. and J. A. Perman. "Current concepts in lactose malabsorption and intolerance." *Journal of the American Dietetic Association* 9: 475, 1989.

Spiller, G. A. (ed). *Dietary Fiber in Human Nutrition,* 2nd ed. Boca Raton: CRC Press, 1993.

Spiller, G. A. and R. Hubbard. *Nutrition Secrets of the Ancients.* Rocklin: Prima Publishing, 1996.

Spiller, G. A., and B. Bruce. *The Cancer Survivor's Nutrition and Health Guide.* Rocklin: Prima Publishing, 1997.

Spiller, G. A. *The Super Pyramid Eating Program.* New York: Times Books, 1993.

United States Department of Agriculture. *Handbook 8-1. Composition of Foods—Dairy and Egg Products . . . Raw, Processed, Prepared.* Washington, DC: USDA, 1976.

Chapter 10: *Understanding Calcium Supplements*

American Dietetic Association. "Position of the American Dietetic Association: vitamin and mineral supplementation." *Journal of the American Dietetic Association* 96: 73, 1996.

Cook, J., S. Dassenko, and P. Whittaker. "Calcium supplementation: effect on iron absorption." *American Journal of Clinical Nutrition* 53: 106, 1991.

Fleming, K. H. and J. T. Heimbach. "Consumption of calcium in the U.S.: food sources and intake levels." *Journal of Nutrition* 124 (Suppl.): S1426, 1994.

Heaney, R. P., K. T. Smith, R. R. Recker, and S. M. Hinders. "Meal effects on calcium absorption." *American Journal of Clinical Nutrition* 49: 372, 1989.

Heaney, R. P., C. M. Weaver, and M. L. Fitzsimmons. "Influence of calcium load on absorption fraction." *Journal of Bone Mineral Research* 5: 1135, 1990.

Lewis, N., Marcus, M., Behling, A., and Greger, J. "Calcium supplements and milk: effects on acid–base balance and on retention of calcium, magnesium, and phosphorus." *American Journal of Clinical Nutrition* 49: 527, 1989.

Nicar, M. J. and C.Y.C. Pak. "Calcium bioavailability from calcium carbonate and calcium citrate." *Journal of Clinical Endocrinology Metabolism* 61: 391, 1985.

Recker, R. R. "Calcium absorption and achlorhydria." *The New England Journal of Medicine* 313: 70, 1985.

Shangaw, R. F. "Factors to consider in the selection of a calcium supplement: proceedings of the 1987 special topic conference on osteoporosis." *Public Health Reports* 104: 46, 1989.

Sheikh, M. and J. Fordtran. "Calcium bioavailability from two calcium carbonate supplements." *The New England Journal of Medicine* 323: 921, 1990.

Whiting, S. "The inhibitory effect of dietary calcium on iron bioavailability: a cause for concern?" *Nutrition Reviews* 53: 77, 1995.

Wood, R. and Zheng, J. "High dietary calcium intakes reduce zinc absorption and balance in humans." *American Journal of Clinical Nutrition* 65: 1803, 1997.

Index